LOW FODMAP ENDOMETRIOSIS COOKBOOK

FOR BEGINNERS

Simple, Delicious Recipes to Ease Symptoms and Nourish Your Body

Kingsley Klopp

To show our appreciation for your purchase, we're delighted to offer you these special bonuses as a heartfelt thank you.

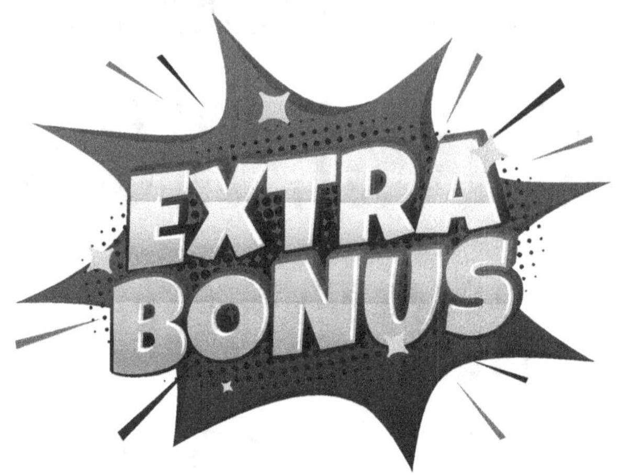

1. A Meal Planner Journal
2. Downloadable E-BOOK featuring full-color images of finished recipes

Table of Contents

Important Note

We are thrilled to accompany you as you explore the potential of the Low FODMAP diet to bring relief and joy into your life. As you set out on this dietary journey, it's important to remember that each individual's body and health needs are unique. While the recipes in this book are designed to be beneficial for many, it's essential to adjust them based on your personal needs and preferences. What works well for one person may not be suitable for another, and that's perfectly okay.

We encourage you to listen to your body and observe how it responds to different foods and recipes. This process of self-discovery is vital in managing endometriosis effectively. If you encounter any uncertainties or if certain recipes do not seem to suit your needs, please do not hesitate to consult with your healthcare provider. Your doctor or a registered dietitian can offer personalized advice and help you tailor the Low FODMAP diet to your specific circumstances.

Additionally, please be aware that the nutritional information provided in this book is approximate and may vary depending on the specific ingredients you use. Variations in product brands, preparation methods, and ingredient substitutions can all affect the nutritional content of a dish. While we strive to offer accurate and helpful nutritional guidance, these figures should be used as a general reference rather than an exact measurement.

Our goal is to empower you with the knowledge and tools to make informed choices about your diet, but it's crucial to approach these changes with flexibility and an open mind. Your well-being is our top priority, and we want to ensure that your experience with the Low FODMAP diet is both positive and effective. Remember, you are not alone on this journey. Many others are navigating similar paths, and there is a community of support and resources available to you. Trust in your ability to find what works best for you, and don't be afraid to seek guidance along the way.

Furthermore, If our cookbook has brought joy to your kitchen and table, we'd be thrilled to hear about your experiences in an Amazon review. On the flip side, if you stumble upon any hiccups while exploring our recipes, don't hesitate to get in touch at **kloppkingsley@gmail.com.** We're here to support your cooking journey every step of the way.

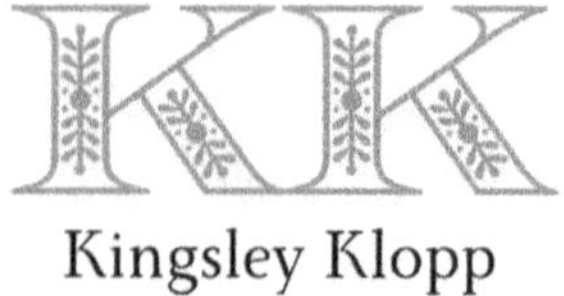

Kingsley Klopp

Introduction

Endometriosis is a condition that affects millions of women worldwide, causing chronic pain, fatigue, and a myriad of other debilitating symptoms. For those living with endometriosis, each day can be a struggle, not just due to the physical pain, but also because of the emotional and mental toll it takes. If you're reading this book, it's likely that you or someone you love is seeking relief from this relentless condition. Welcome to **Low FODMAP Endometriosis Cookbook for Beginners,**" where we explore a path to managing your symptoms and reclaiming your quality of life through the power of nutrition.The journey to finding relief from endometriosis often feels like navigating a maze, with many dead ends and few clear paths. Traditional treatments such as surgery and hormone therapy may offer some relief but often come with significant side effects and are not always effective for everyone. This is where dietary changes, specifically the Low FODMAP diet, come into play. Scientific research and anecdotal evidence suggest that diet can have a profound impact on endometriosis symptoms, offering a natural and holistic approach to managing this condition. The Low FODMAP diet, originally designed to alleviate symptoms of irritable bowel syndrome (IBS), has shown promise in reducing the gastrointestinal distress that many endometriosis sufferers experience.

FODMAPs are short-chain carbohydrates that are poorly absorbed in the small intestine, leading to fermentation and the production of gas when they reach the colon. For those with endometriosis, this can exacerbate symptoms such as bloating, abdominal pain, and discomfort. By following a Low FODMAP diet, you can minimize these triggers and create a more stable, manageable digestive environment. This cookbook is not just a collection of recipes; it is a comprehensive guide to understanding and implementing the Low FODMAP diet specifically tailored for endometriosis sufferers. We have carefully curated recipes that are not only delicious but also designed to support your health and wellbeing. Each recipe is crafted to be simple, nutritious, and aligned with Low FODMAP principles, making it easy for you to prepare meals that nourish your body and help reduce your symptoms. Embarking on a new dietary regimen can be daunting, especially when you are already dealing with the challenges of endometriosis. This book aims to make the transition as smooth as possible. We start with an in-depth explanation of what endometriosis is, how the Low FODMAP diet works, and why it can be beneficial for managing your symptoms. From there, we guide you through meal planning, grocery shopping, and preparing your kitchen for success. Each chapter is designed to provide you with the knowledge, tools, and confidence you need to take control of your diet and, ultimately, your health.

But this book is about more than just food. It is about hope and empowerment. It is about finding a sense of control in the face of a condition that often leaves you feeling powerless. It is about discovering that you have the ability to make choices that positively impact your life. By choosing to nourish your body with the right foods, you are taking a proactive step towards managing your endometriosis and improving your quality of life.

We invite you to join us on this journey to better health. Let **Low FODMAP Endometriosis Cookbook for Beginners** be your guide and companion as you explore the potential of the Low FODMAP diet to bring relief, comfort, and joy back into your life. Together, we can navigate the complexities of endometriosis and find a path to a healthier, happier you.

Understanding Endometriosis

What is Endometriosis?

Endometriosis is a chronic, often debilitating condition that affects millions of women worldwide, yet remains largely misunderstood and under-discussed. At its core, endometriosis involves the growth of tissue similar to the lining inside the uterus, known as the endometrium, outside the uterine cavity. This rogue tissue can be found on the ovaries, fallopian tubes, the outer surface of the uterus, and other organs within the pelvis. Imagine the agony of enduring relentless pain month after month, the kind that disrupts your daily life and steals moments of joy. This is the harsh reality for many women with endometriosis. The misplaced endometrial-like tissue continues to act as it would inside the uterus – it thickens, breaks down, and bleeds with each menstrual cycle. But unlike the tissue in the uterus, which leaves the body during menstruation, this blood has no way to escape. The result is inflammation, scar tissue, and adhesions, which are bands of fibrous tissue that can cause organs to stick together. The symptoms of endometriosis can be as varied as the women it affects, but they often include severe pelvic pain, especially during menstruation. This pain can be so intense that it overshadows everything else, making it difficult to concentrate, work, or enjoy life. Some women also experience pain during intercourse, bowel movements, or urination. The constant fatigue and gastrointestinal issues like bloating, diarrhea, and constipation add another layer of distress.

Endometriosis doesn't just impact physical health; it also takes a significant emotional toll. The chronic pain and unpredictable flare-ups can lead to anxiety and depression. Relationships can suffer as intimacy becomes painful and plans are often disrupted by sudden bouts of pain. Many women feel isolated and misunderstood, as the invisible nature of their pain makes it hard for others to comprehend the extent of their suffering. One of the most heartbreaking aspects of endometriosis is its impact on fertility. Up to 40% of women with infertility issues are found to have endometriosis. The condition can damage the ovaries, block fallopian tubes, and create a hostile environment for egg fertilization and embryo implantation. The journey to motherhood becomes fraught with uncertainty, adding another layer of emotional pain.

Despite being one of the most common gynecological conditions, endometriosis is often misdiagnosed or overlooked. On average, it takes about 7 to 10 years from the onset of symptoms for a woman to receive a correct diagnosis. This delay can be attributed to a lack of awareness among healthcare providers and the normalization of menstrual pain in society. Women are often told that their pain is just part of being a woman and are not taken seriously until the condition has significantly progressed. The path to managing endometriosis is challenging and often involves a combination of treatments. Pain relief can be achieved through medications, hormonal therapies, and in some cases, surgery. However, these treatments are not cures, and many women continue to struggle with symptoms throughout their lives.

Living with endometriosis requires immense strength and resilience. Each day is a testament to the determination and courage of those affected, as they navigate a world that often fails to see their invisible battles. It's time for greater awareness, empathy, and research to ensure that no woman has to suffer in silence or wait years for relief. Endometriosis is not just a condition; it's a profound and life-altering experience that demands our attention and compassion.

Symptoms and Diagnosis

Symptoms of Endometriosis
The symptoms of endometriosis can vary greatly, but they often begin with one of the most common and debilitating indicators: **chronic pelvic pain**. This pain typically intensifies during menstruation, turning what should be a natural, albeit uncomfortable, part of a woman's life into an agonizing ordeal. The pain can be so severe that it disrupts daily activities, making it difficult to work, study, or even move.

Pain during intercourse is another distressing symptom. For many women, what should be an intimate and loving experience becomes a source of anxiety and discomfort. This can strain relationships and lead to emotional distress, compounding the physical pain with feelings of isolation and frustration. Women with endometriosis often experience **painful bowel movements or urination**, particularly during their periods. This can lead to a fear of basic bodily functions, creating a constant state of anxiety and dread. Additionally, many women suffer from **gastrointestinal issues** like bloating, diarrhea, constipation, and nausea, often leading to misdiagnoses such as irritable bowel syndrome (IBS).

Another common and emotionally devastating symptom is **infertility**. For women dreaming of motherhood, the struggle to conceive can be heart-wrenching. Endometriosis can damage the reproductive organs, making natural conception difficult or impossible. The journey through infertility treatments can be long, expensive, and emotionally draining, adding another layer of suffering.
Fatigue is also a frequent companion of endometriosis. Chronic pain and the body's constant battle against inflammation can leave women feeling exhausted, no matter how much rest they get. This relentless fatigue affects every aspect of life, from work performance to social interactions, often leading to a sense of helplessness and frustration.

Diagnosis of Endometriosis
The path to a diagnosis of endometriosis is often long and fraught with challenges. On average, it takes **7 to 10 years** from the onset of symptoms for a woman to receive an accurate diagnosis. This delay is due to a combination of factors, including a lack of awareness among healthcare providers, the normalization of menstrual pain, and the variable nature of the symptoms.

The journey often begins with multiple visits to doctors, each offering different explanations for the pain. Women are frequently told that their pain is normal or psychosomatic, leading to feelings of disbelief and self-doubt. This dismissal can be one of the most emotionally taxing parts of the endometriosis experience.

Imaging tests such as ultrasounds and MRIs are often used, but they can miss smaller endometrial lesions, leading to false negatives. The definitive diagnosis of endometriosis usually requires a **laparoscopy**, a surgical procedure in which a camera is inserted into the pelvic cavity to directly visualize and sometimes biopsy the endometrial tissue. This invasive step can be daunting, but it often brings relief by providing clear answers and paving the way for targeted treatment. Receiving a diagnosis can be a double-edged sword: it brings validation and the possibility of effective treatment, but it also confirms a chronic condition that requires lifelong management. The emotional impact of this diagnosis is profound. It can bring a sense of relief, but also fear and uncertainty about the future.

The Low FODMAP Diet

What is FODMAP?

The term FODMAP might sound technical and unfamiliar, but for many people suffering from digestive disorders, it represents a crucial concept that can significantly impact their quality of life. FODMAP stands for Fermentable Oligosaccharides, Disaccharides, Monosaccharides, and Polyols – a group of short-chain carbohydrates and sugar alcohols found in various foods. Understanding what FODMAPs are and how they affect the body can be a transformative step toward managing conditions like irritable bowel syndrome (IBS) and even endometriosis, where digestive issues often complicate an already challenging situation.

What are FODMAPs?

FODMAPs are specific types of carbohydrates that some people have difficulty digesting. When consumed, these carbohydrates travel through the stomach and small intestine without being properly absorbed. When they reach the large intestine, they are fermented by gut bacteria, which produces gas and draws water into the colon. This can lead to symptoms like bloating, gas, abdominal pain, diarrhea, and constipation – symptoms that can be particularly severe and disruptive.

Breaking Down FODMAPs

- **Oligosaccharides**: Found in foods like wheat, garlic, onions, and legumes. These are chains of simple sugars that many people struggle to digest.
- **Disaccharides**: The most common disaccharide is lactose, found in dairy products like milk, cheese, and yogurt. Lactose intolerance is a widespread issue, causing bloating, diarrhea, and stomach cramps.
- **Monosaccharides**: Fructose, found in fruits, honey, and high-fructose corn syrup, is a monosaccharide. Some people have difficulty absorbing fructose, leading to digestive distress.
- **Polyols**: These sugar alcohols, including sorbitol and mannitol, are found in certain fruits and vegetables, as well as artificial sweeteners. They can be particularly problematic for sensitive digestive systems.

The Impact of FODMAPs

For someone dealing with digestive issues, consuming high-FODMAP foods can turn a simple meal into a source of agony. Imagine the anticipation of enjoying a favorite dish, only to be met with hours of crippling pain and discomfort afterward. The constant need to scrutinize every food label and menu can make eating a source of anxiety rather than pleasure. This is the reality for many people struggling with FODMAP sensitivity.

The Low FODMAP Diet

The low FODMAP diet, developed by researchers at Monash University in Australia, offers a beacon of hope. It involves three phases:

1. **Elimination**: Removing all high-FODMAP foods from the diet for several weeks to allow the digestive system to calm down.
2. **Reintroduction**: Gradually reintroducing FODMAPs one at a time to identify specific triggers. This step is crucial for personalizing the diet to each individual's tolerance.
3. **Personalization**: Creating a long-term eating plan that avoids high-FODMAP foods that trigger symptoms while including those that don't.

Emotional Journey of Managing FODMAPs

Embarking on a low FODMAP diet can be daunting. It requires significant lifestyle changes, meticulous planning, and often a deep emotional adjustment. There can be a sense of loss and frustration at having to give up beloved foods. Eating out becomes a challenge, and social gatherings can be fraught with anxiety about potential triggers.

However, the potential rewards are life-changing. Finding relief from chronic digestive symptoms can restore a sense of normalcy and well-being. Imagine waking up without the dread of pain and discomfort, enjoying meals without fear, and reclaiming the joy of eating. The journey to understanding and managing FODMAPs is not just about dietary changes; it's about reclaiming control over one's life and health.

Benefits of a Low FODMAP Diet

Living with endometriosis often feels like navigating a maze of pain and uncertainty. The physical agony, coupled with the emotional toll, can make each day a challenge. Among the various approaches to managing this chronic condition, the low FODMAP diet has emerged as a beacon of hope for many. While it was initially designed to alleviate symptoms of irritable bowel syndrome (IBS), research and anecdotal evidence suggest that it can also provide significant relief for those suffering from endometriosis. Understanding the benefits of a low FODMAP diet for endometriosis can be a transformative step towards reclaiming control over one's health and well-being.

Understanding the Connection

Endometriosis and digestive issues often go hand in hand. The inflammation and adhesions caused by endometriosis can affect the intestines, leading to symptoms that mimic IBS, such as bloating, gas, diarrhea, and constipation. These symptoms can exacerbate the pain and discomfort already caused by endometriosis, creating a vicious cycle of suffering. This is where the low FODMAP diet comes into play, offering a potential solution by addressing these gastrointestinal issues directly.

Benefits of a Low FODMAP Diet

1. Reduction in Abdominal Pain

One of the most debilitating aspects of endometriosis is the chronic abdominal pain. The low FODMAP diet helps reduce this pain by minimizing the intake of fermentable carbohydrates that contribute to bloating and gas. By eliminating these triggers, many women find significant relief from the constant, gnawing pain that can dominate their lives. Imagine the sheer relief of waking up without that familiar, unrelenting ache in your belly – it's like a ray of sunshine breaking through a cloudy sky.

2. Decreased Bloating and Gas

Bloating can be more than just uncomfortable; it can be painful and distressing, especially when dealing with endometriosis. The low FODMAP diet reduces bloating by preventing the fermentation of certain carbohydrates in the gut. This can lead to a flatter stomach and less discomfort, making it easier to move, breathe, and engage in daily activities without the constant feeling of being weighed down.

3. Improved Bowel Habits

Endometriosis can wreak havoc on bowel habits, causing constipation, diarrhea, or a frustrating mix of both. The low FODMAP diet can help normalize bowel movements by eliminating foods that irritate the gut. For many women, this means fewer frantic dashes to the bathroom and less time spent feeling uncomfortable or in pain. Regular, predictable bowel movements can restore a sense of normalcy and control, reducing anxiety and improving quality of life.

4. Enhanced Energy Levels
Chronic pain and digestive issues can sap energy, leaving those with endometriosis feeling perpetually exhausted. By alleviating gastrointestinal symptoms, the low FODMAP diet can help restore energy levels. When the body isn't constantly fighting inflammation and discomfort, it can use its resources more efficiently, leading to improved stamina and vitality. Imagine the joy of feeling energized enough to pursue passions, engage with loved ones, and live life to the fullest.

5. Better Mental Health
The constant pain and discomfort of endometriosis can take a severe toll on mental health, leading to feelings of anxiety, depression, and isolation. Relief from gastrointestinal symptoms can have a profound impact on emotional well-being. Feeling physically better can boost mood, enhance mental clarity, and foster a more positive outlook on life. The journey to managing endometriosis is not just about reducing physical pain but also about finding peace and happiness.

Hence, the low FODMAP diet offers a promising approach to managing the complex and often intertwined symptoms of endometriosis and digestive issues. By reducing abdominal pain, bloating, and improving bowel habits, it can significantly enhance the quality of life for those affected. Beyond the physical benefits, it also brings emotional relief, offering hope and a path to a more manageable, fulfilling life. For anyone living with endometriosis, exploring the low FODMAP diet could be a transformative step toward reclaiming their health and happiness.

How to Follow a Low FODMAP Diet

Setting out on a low FODMAP diet can feel overwhelming at first, but understanding the steps and the reasons behind them can make the journey much smoother. This diet, designed to manage gastrointestinal symptoms, requires careful planning and commitment. However, the rewards of reduced pain, discomfort, and a better quality of life make it worth the effort. Here's a comprehensive guide on how to follow a low FODMAP diet, infused with empathy and encouragement to help you navigate this path.

Understanding the Low FODMAP Diet

The low FODMAP diet involves three phases: elimination, reintroduction, and personalization. Each phase is crucial for identifying and managing your unique food triggers.

Phase 1: Elimination

The first phase is the elimination phase, where high FODMAP foods are removed from your diet. This phase typically lasts between four to six weeks and aims to reduce symptoms by minimizing the intake of fermentable carbohydrates.

Steps to Follow:

1. **Educate Yourself**: Learn about high FODMAP foods to avoid. These include certain fruits (like apples and pears), vegetables (such as onions and garlic), dairy products (like milk and soft cheeses), and sweeteners (such as honey and high-fructose corn syrup).
2. **Plan Your Meals**: Create meal plans that include low FODMAP foods. Lean proteins, lactose-free dairy, most nuts and seeds, and certain fruits (such as strawberries and blueberries) are good options. Online resources and cookbooks can provide recipes to keep your meals varied and enjoyable.
3. **Read Labels Carefully**: Processed foods often contain hidden high FODMAP ingredients. Reading labels meticulously helps avoid unintentional consumption of these ingredients.
4. **Keep a Food Diary**: Track what you eat and any symptoms you experience. This will help identify patterns and make it easier to pinpoint problem foods later.

Phase 2: Reintroduction

Once your symptoms have improved, you move to the reintroduction phase. This phase helps identify specific FODMAPs that trigger your symptoms.

Steps to Follow:

1. **Introduce One FODMAP at a Time**: Gradually reintroduce high FODMAP foods, one group at a time (e.g., oligosaccharides, disaccharides, monosaccharides, and polyols). Start with a small amount and gradually increase it while monitoring your symptoms.
2. **Monitor and Record**: Keep detailed notes on your symptoms during each reintroduction. This will help determine which FODMAPs are problematic and which are well-tolerated.
3. **Consult a Dietitian**: A dietitian can provide guidance and support during this phase, helping you interpret your reactions and adjust your diet accordingly.

Phase 3: Personalization

The final phase is personalization, where you create a long-term eating plan tailored to your individual tolerance levels. This phase aims to maintain symptom relief while expanding your diet to include as many foods as possible.

Steps to Follow:

1. **Develop a Balanced Diet**: Incorporate a wide variety of low and moderate FODMAP foods to ensure nutritional balance and enjoyment.
2. **Stay Flexible**: Your tolerance to FODMAPs may change over time. Regularly reassess your diet and symptoms, and be prepared to make adjustments as needed.
3. **Practice Mindful Eating**: Pay attention to how your body responds to different foods and situations. Stress and other factors can influence symptoms, so holistic management is essential.

Emotional Support and Self-Care

Following a low FODMAP diet can be emotionally challenging. It requires discipline and sometimes involves significant lifestyle changes. Here are some tips to help you manage the emotional aspects:

1. **Seek Support**: Connect with others who are following the same diet. Online forums, support groups, and social media communities can offer encouragement, tips, and shared experiences.
2. **Celebrate Small Wins**: Recognize and celebrate improvements in your symptoms, no matter how small. Each step forward is progress.
3. **Be Patient and Compassionate**: Understand that this journey takes time. Be kind to yourself during setbacks and celebrate your successes.
4. **Involve Loved Ones**: Share your dietary needs with family and friends. Their understanding and support can make social situations less stressful and more enjoyable.

Foods to Avoid and Foods to Enjoy

Foods to Avoid

High FODMAP foods are those that contain fermentable oligosaccharides, disaccharides, monosaccharides, and polyols. These are the carbohydrates that can exacerbate digestive symptoms.

Oligosaccharides

- **Fructans**: Found in wheat, onions, garlic, and certain vegetables like asparagus, leeks, and broccoli.
- **Galactans**: Present in legumes such as beans, lentils, chickpeas, and soy products.

Disaccharides

- **Lactose**: Found in dairy products like milk, soft cheeses, yogurt, and ice cream. Many people with FODMAP sensitivities cannot properly digest lactose.

Monosaccharides

- **Fructose**: Present in high amounts in fruits such as apples, pears, mangoes, and watermelon, as well as in honey and high-fructose corn syrup.

Polyols

- **Sorbitol and Mannitol**: Found in certain fruits (like apples, pears, and stone fruits) and vegetables (such as mushrooms and cauliflower), as well as in sugar-free gums and candies.

Common High FODMAP Foods to Avoid

- **Wheat-based products**: Bread, pasta, cereals, crackers, and baked goods.
- **Certain fruits**: Apples, pears, mangoes, cherries, and watermelon.
- **Certain vegetables**: Onions, garlic, asparagus, cauliflower, and mushrooms.
- **Dairy products**: Milk, soft cheeses, yogurt, and ice cream.
- **Legumes and pulses**: Beans, lentils, chickpeas, and soy products.
- **Sweeteners**: Honey, high-fructose corn syrup, and sugar alcohols (such as sorbitol and mannitol).

Foods to Enjoy

While the list of high FODMAP foods might seem extensive, there are plenty of delicious and nutritious low FODMAP options to include in your diet. These foods are easier to digest and less likely to cause uncomfortable symptoms.

Fruits

- **Low FODMAP Fruits**: Bananas, blueberries, strawberries, oranges, grapes, kiwi, and pineapple. These fruits are generally well-tolerated in moderate amounts.

Vegetables

- **Low FODMAP Vegetables**: Carrots, spinach, kale, zucchini, cucumbers, bell peppers, tomatoes, and potatoes. These vegetables can be enjoyed raw, cooked, or in a variety of dishes.

Grains and Cereals
- **Gluten-Free Grains**: Rice, quinoa, oats, millet, and polenta. These grains are not only low FODMAP but also provide essential nutrients and fiber.
- **Low FODMAP Bread and Pasta**: Gluten-free bread and pasta options made from rice, corn, or quinoa.

Proteins
- **Meat and Poultry**: Beef, pork, chicken, turkey, and lamb. These proteins are naturally low FODMAP when prepared without high FODMAP marinades or sauces.
- **Seafood**: Fish, shrimp, and other shellfish. Fresh seafood is a great source of lean protein.
- **Eggs**: Eggs are versatile and can be included in various meals.

Dairy Alternatives
- **Lactose-Free Dairy**: Lactose-free milk, cheese, and yogurt. These products provide the benefits of dairy without the discomfort.
- **Plant-Based Milks**: Almond milk, coconut milk, and rice milk (ensure they are low FODMAP and unsweetened).

Nuts and Seeds
- **Low FODMAP Nuts and Seeds**: Almonds (in limited amounts), walnuts, macadamia nuts, chia seeds, and pumpkin seeds. These are great for snacking or adding to dishes for extra crunch.

Condiments and Flavorings
- **Herbs and Spices**: Basil, oregano, thyme, rosemary, and ginger. These can enhance the flavor of meals without adding FODMAPs.
- **Low FODMAP Condiments**: Mustard, mayonnaise, and soy sauce (in small amounts). Check labels to ensure they do not contain high FODMAP ingredients.

Creating a Balanced Diet

While it's essential to avoid high FODMAP foods to manage symptoms, it's equally important to ensure your diet remains balanced and nutritious. Incorporate a variety of low FODMAP foods to meet your nutritional needs and keep your meals interesting and satisfying.

Meal Planning Tips
- **Variety is Key**: Rotate different fruits, vegetables, proteins, and grains to ensure you get a wide range of nutrients.
- **Experiment with Recipes**: Look for low FODMAP cookbooks and online resources to find new recipes and meal ideas. This can make the diet more enjoyable and less restrictive.
- **Preparation and Planning**: Plan your meals and snacks ahead of time to avoid the temptation of high FODMAP convenience foods. Prepare meals in advance to make sticking to the diet easier, especially during busy times.

Special Note

Let us reiterate, While the recipes in this book are designed to be beneficial for many, it's essential to adjust them based on your personal needs and preferences. What works well for one person may not be suitable for another, and that's perfectly okay. We encourage you to listen to your body and observe how it responds to different foods and recipes. This process of self-discovery is vital in managing endometriosis effectively. If you encounter any uncertainties or if certain recipes do not seem to suit your needs, please do not hesitate to consult with your healthcare provider. Your doctor or a registered dietitian can offer personalized advice and help you tailor the Low FODMAP diet to your specific circumstances. Additionally, please be aware that the nutritional information provided in this book is approximate and may vary depending on the specific ingredients you use. Variations in product brands, preparation methods, and ingredient substitutions can all affect the nutritional content of a dish. While we strive to offer accurate and helpful nutritional guidance, these figures should be used as a general reference rather than an exact measurement.

Breakfast Recipes

1. Sweet Potato Toast
Ingredients
- 1 large sweet potato
- 1 tablespoon olive oil
- 1 avocado, mashed
- 1 teaspoon lemon juice
- 1 teaspoon chili flakes (optional)
- 1 egg (optional for protein)
- 1 teaspoon chives, chopped

Instructions
1. Preheat your oven to 400°F (200°C).
2. Wash and peel the sweet potato. Cut it into 1/4-inch thick slices lengthwise.
3. Brush both sides of the sweet potato slices with olive oil.
4. Place the slices on a baking sheet lined with parchment paper.
5. Bake for 20-25 minutes, flipping halfway through, until tender and slightly crispy.
6. While the sweet potato is baking, mash the avocado in a bowl and mix with lemon juice and chili flakes.
7. Optionally, cook the egg to your liking (boiled, poached, or scrambled).
8. Once the sweet potato slices are done, let them cool slightly. Spread the avocado mixture on top and add the egg if using. Garnish with chopped chives.

Nutrition Info per Serving
- Calories: 220
- Protein: 3g
- Carbohydrates: 22g
- Fat: 14g
- Fiber: 7g

Serves
- 2

Cooking Time
- 30 minutes

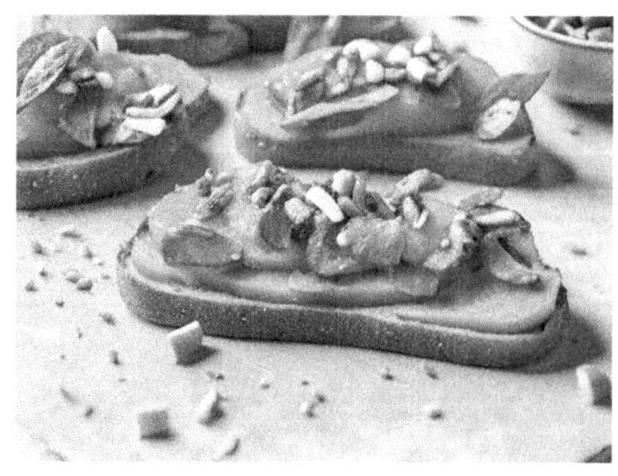

2. Rice-Based Cereal

Ingredients

- 1 cup rice flakes (gluten-free)
- 2 cups lactose-free milk or almond milk
- 1 tablespoon chia seeds
- 1 tablespoon maple syrup
- 1/2 teaspoon cinnamon
- 1/4 cup blueberries

Instructions

1. In a medium saucepan, combine rice flakes and milk. Bring to a boil over medium heat.
2. Reduce heat and simmer for about 5 minutes, stirring occasionally, until the cereal thickens.
3. Stir in chia seeds, maple syrup, and cinnamon.
4. Cook for another 2-3 minutes, stirring constantly.
5. Remove from heat and let it sit for a few minutes to thicken further.
6. Serve topped with blueberries.

Nutrition Info per Serving

- Calories: 190
- Protein: 5g
- Carbohydrates: 36g
- Fat: 4g
- Fiber: 4g

Serves

- 2

Cooking Time

- 10 minutes

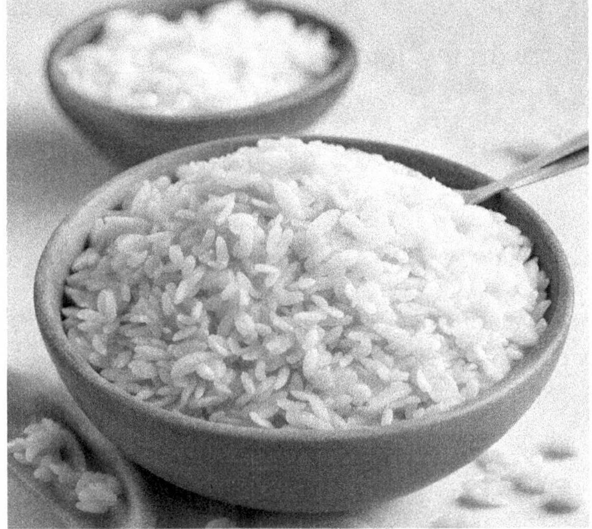

3. Stir-Fried Tempeh

Ingredients

- 1 cup tempeh, cubed
- 1 tablespoon olive oil
- 1/2 red bell pepper, diced
- 1/2 cup spinach, chopped
- 1 tablespoon low-sodium soy sauce
- 1 teaspoon ginger, grated
- 1 teaspoon sesame seeds

Instructions

1. Heat olive oil in a non-stick pan over medium heat.
2. Add cubed tempeh and cook for about 5-7 minutes until golden brown, stirring occasionally.
3. Add diced red bell pepper and cook for another 3-4 minutes until tender.
4. Add chopped spinach, soy sauce, and grated ginger. Cook for another 2-3 minutes until spinach is wilted.
5. Serve immediately, garnished with sesame seeds.

Nutrition Info per Serving

- Calories: 220
- Protein: 12g
- Carbohydrates: 10g
- Fat: 16g
- Fiber: 5g

Serves

- 2

Cooking Time

- 15 minutes

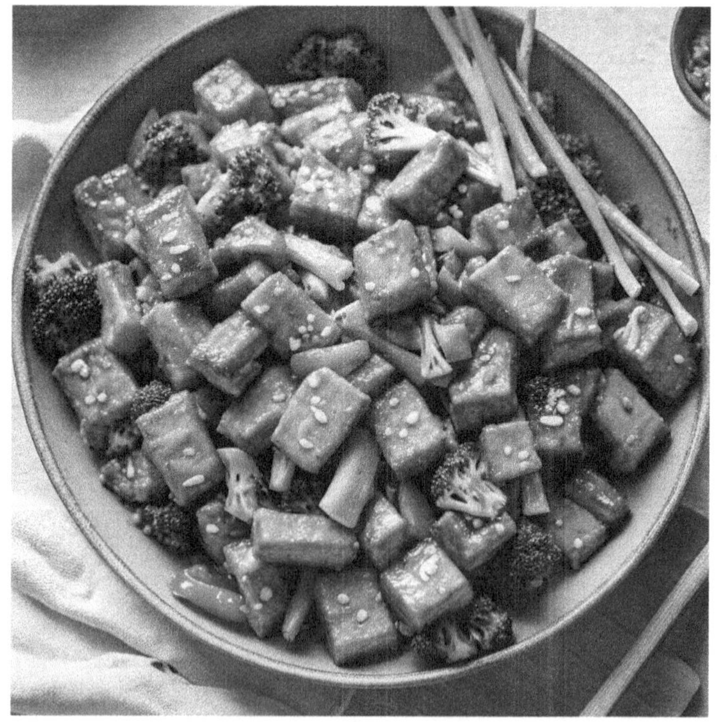

4. Homemade Hash Browns

Ingredients

- 2 large potatoes, peeled and grated
- 1 tablespoon olive oil
- 1/2 teaspoon paprika
- 1/2 teaspoon garlic-infused oil
- 1 tablespoon chives, chopped

Instructions

1. Rinse grated potatoes under cold water to remove excess starch. Pat dry with paper towels.
2. Heat olive oil in a large skillet over medium-high heat.
3. Add grated potatoes, pressing them into an even layer. Cook for 5-7 minutes until the bottom is golden brown.
4. Flip the hash browns and cook for another 5-7 minutes until the other side is golden and crispy.
5. Remove from heat and transfer to a plate. Drizzle with garlic-infused oil and sprinkle with paprika and chopped chives.

Nutrition Info per Serving

- Calories: 160
- Protein: 2g
- Carbohydrates: 24g
- Fat: 7g
- Fiber: 3g

Serves

- 2

Cooking Time

- 20 minutes

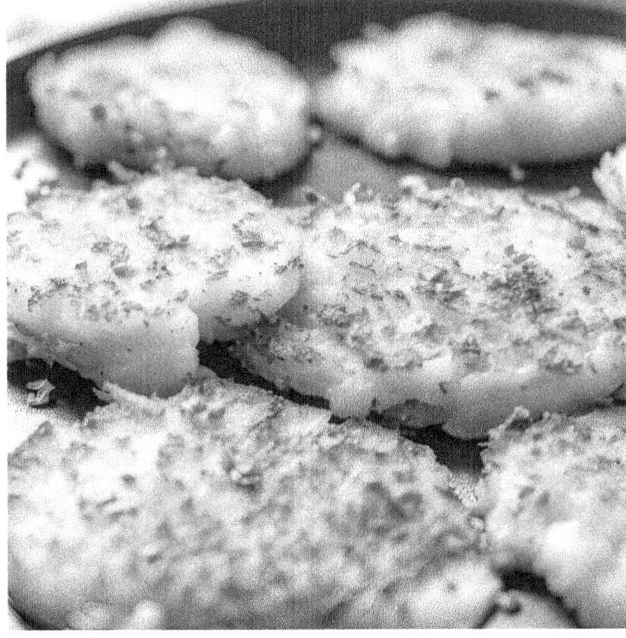

5. Almond Flour Muffins

Ingredients

- 2 cups almond flour
- 1/4 teaspoon baking soda
- 1/4 teaspoon salt
- 1/4 cup maple syrup
- 2 large eggs
- 1 teaspoon vanilla extract
- 1/4 cup lactose-free yogurt or coconut yogurt
- 1/4 cup blueberries (optional)

Instructions

1. Preheat your oven to 350°F (175°C). Line a muffin tin with paper liners.
2. In a large bowl, combine almond flour, baking soda, and salt.
3. In a separate bowl, whisk together maple syrup, eggs, vanilla extract, and yogurt until smooth.
4. Pour the wet ingredients into the dry ingredients and mix until just combined.
5. Fold in blueberries if using.
6. Divide the batter evenly among the muffin cups.
7. Bake for 20-25 minutes, until a toothpick inserted into the center comes out clean.
8. Allow muffins to cool in the tin for 5 minutes before transferring to a wire rack to cool completely.

Nutrition Info per Serving

- Calories: 180
- Protein: 6g
- Carbohydrates: 12g
- Fat: 13g
- Fiber: 3g

Serves

- 8 muffins

Cooking Time

- 30 minutes

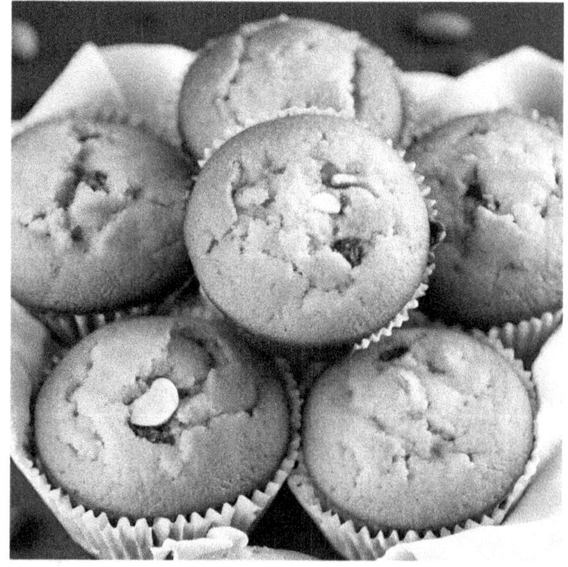

6. Buckwheat Crepes

Ingredients

- 1 cup buckwheat flour
- 1 1/4 cups lactose-free milk or almond milk
- 2 large eggs
- 1 tablespoon olive oil (plus more for cooking)
- 1 teaspoon vanilla extract
- 1 tablespoon maple syrup (optional for sweet crepes)

Instructions

1. In a mixing bowl, whisk together buckwheat flour, milk, eggs, olive oil, and vanilla extract until smooth. If making sweet crepes, add the maple syrup.
2. Heat a non-stick skillet over medium heat and lightly grease with olive oil.
3. Pour abo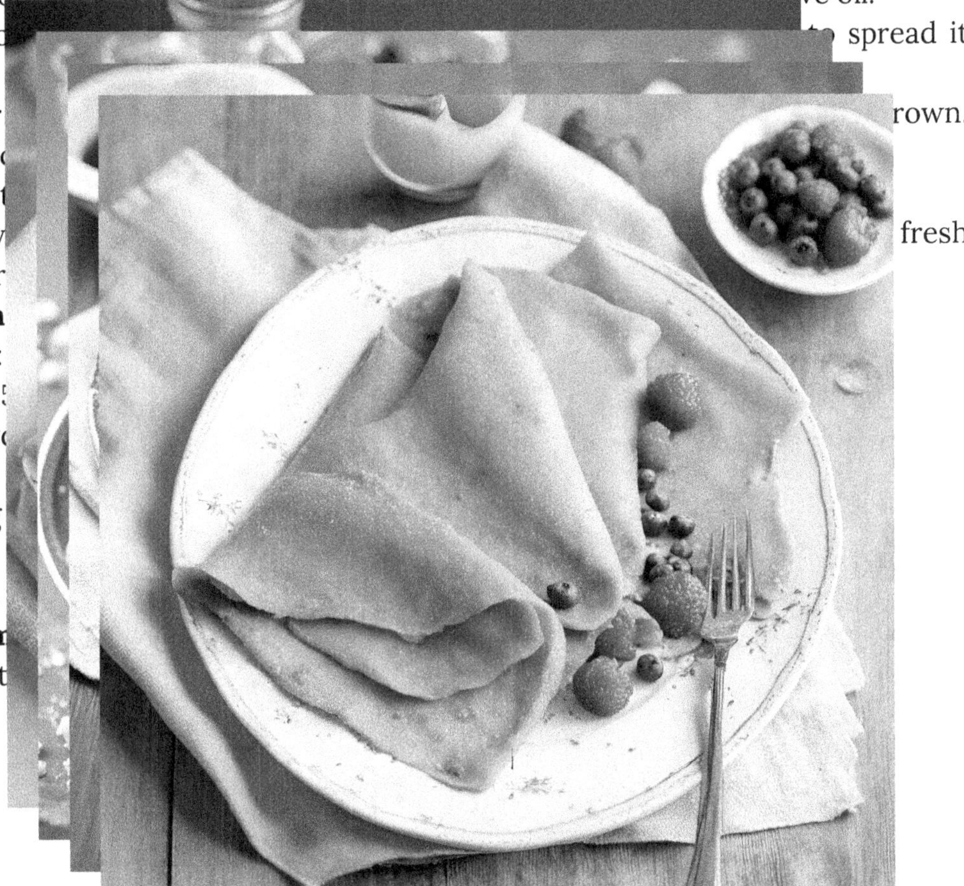 spread it evenly.
4. Cook for rown. Flip and
5. Remove
6. Serve w fresh strawber

Nutrition In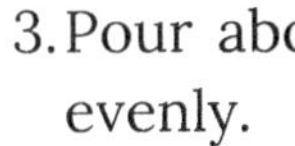

- Calories:
- Protein:
- Carbohy
- Fat: 4g
- Fiber: 2g

Serves

- 4 crepes

Cooking Tim

- 20 minut

7. Grilled Plantains

Ingredients

- 2 ripe plantains
- 1 tablespoon olive oil
- 1 teaspoon cinnamon

Instructions

1. Preheat a grill or grill pan over medium-high heat.
2. Peel the plantains and slice them diagonally into 1/2-inch thick pieces.
3. Brush both sides of the plantain slices with olive oil.
4. Place the plantain slices on the grill and cook for 3-4 minutes on each side, until grill marks appear and the plantains are tender.
5. Sprinkle with cinnamon before serving.

Nutrition Info per Serving

- Calories: 180
- Protein: 1g
- Carbohydrates: 31g
- Fat: 7g
- Fiber: 2g

Serves

- 2

Cooking Time

- 10 minutes

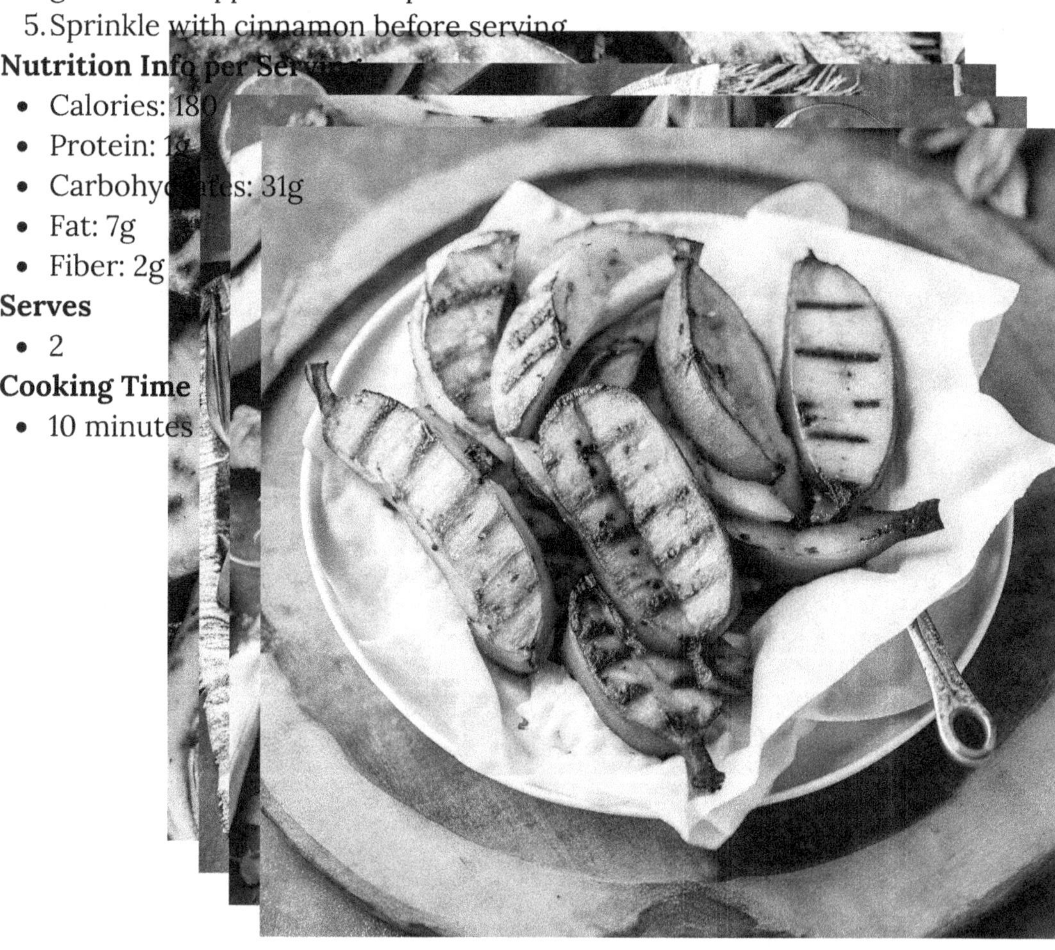

8. Potato and Carrot Rosti

Ingredients

- 2 large potatoes, peeled and grated
- 1 large carrot, peeled and grated
- 2 tablespoons olive oil
- 1 tablespoon chives, chopped

Instructions

1. Preheat the oven to 400°F (200°C).
2. Place the grated potatoes and carrot in a clean kitchen towel and squeeze out excess moisture.
3. In a large bowl, mix the grated potatoes and carrot.
4. Heat 1 tablespoon of olive oil in an oven-safe skillet over medium heat.
5. Add the potato and carrot mixture to the skillet, pressing it down firmly.
6. Cook for 5-7 minutes until the bottom is golden brown.
7. Flip the rosti and transfer the skillet to the oven. Bake for 15-20 minutes until crispy and golden.
8. Garnish with chopped chives before serving.

Nutrition Info per Serving

- Calories: 150
- Protein: 2g
- Carbohydrates: 20g
- Fat: 7g
- Fiber: 3g

Serves

- 2

Cooking Time

- 30 minutes

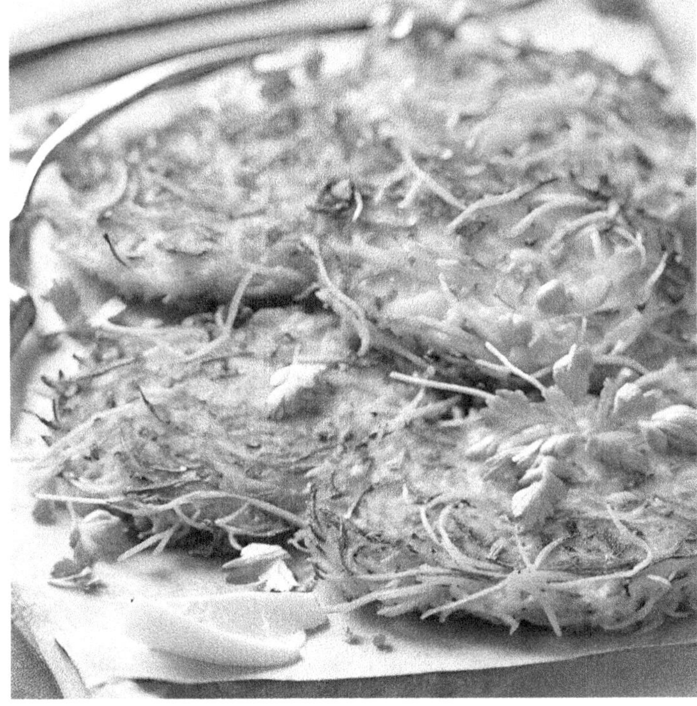

9. Sourdough Toast

Ingredients

- 4 slices sourdough bread
- 1 avocado, mashed
- 1 tablespoon lemon juice
- 1 teaspoon chili flakes (optional)
- 2 tablespoons olive oil
- 1 teaspoon chives, chopped

Instructions

1. Toast the sourdough bread slices until golden brown.
2. In a bowl, mash the avocado and mix with lemon juice and chili flakes.
3. Drizzle the toasted sourdough bread with olive oil.
4. Spread the avocado mixture on each slice of toast.
5. Garnish with chopped chives before serving.

Nutrition Info per Serving

- Calories: 220
- Protein: 5g
- Carbohydrates: 30g
- Fat: 10g
- Fiber: 5g

Serves

- 2

Cooking Time

- 10 minutes

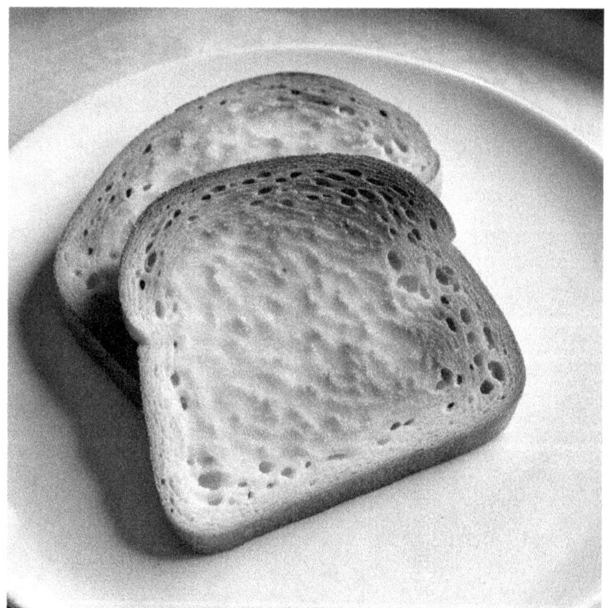

10. Quinoa Porridge

Ingredients

- 1 cup quinoa, rinsed
- 2 cups lactose-free milk or almond milk
- 1 tablespoon maple syrup
- 1/2 teaspoon cinnamon
- 1/4 cup blueberries
- 1 tablespoon chia seeds

Instructions

1. In a medium saucepan, combine quinoa and milk. Bring to a boil over medium heat.
2. Reduce heat and simmer for about 15 minutes, stirring occasionally, until the quinoa is tender and the liquid is absorbed.
3. Stir in maple syrup and cinnamon.
4. Remove from heat and let it sit for a few minutes to thicken.
5. Serve topped with blueberries and chia seeds.

Nutrition Info per Serving

- Calories: 250
- Protein: 8g
- Carbohydrates: 38g
- Fat: 7g
- Fiber: 5g

Serves

- 2

Cooking Time

- 20 minutes

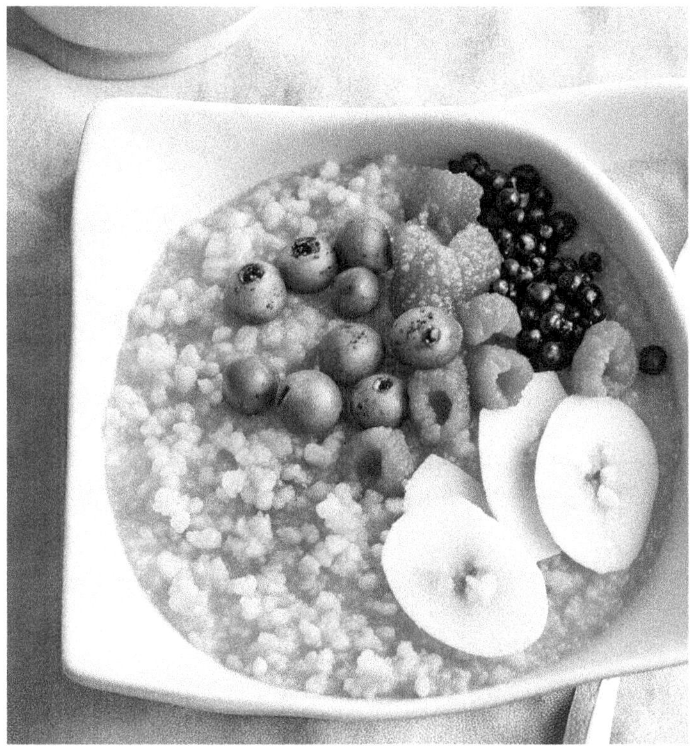

11. Buckwheat Pancakes

Ingredients

- 1 cup buckwheat flour
- 1 tablespoon sugar
- 1 teaspoon baking powder
- 1/2 teaspoon baking soda
- 1 cup lactose-free milk or almond milk
- 1 large egg
- 2 tablespoons melted coconut oil
- 1 teaspoon vanilla extract

Instructions

1. In a large bowl, mix together buckwheat flour, sugar, baking powder, and baking soda.
2. In another bowl, whisk together the milk, egg, melted coconut oil, and vanilla extract.
3. Pour the wet ingredients into the dry ingredients and stir until just combined.
4. Heat a non-stick skillet over medium heat and lightly grease with coconut oil.
5. Pour 1/4 cup of batter onto the skillet for each pancake. Cook until bubbles form on the surface, then flip and cook until golden brown.
6. Serve warm with maple syrup and fresh berries.

Nutrition Info per Serving

- Calories: 160
- Protein: 5g
- Carbohydrates: 20g
- Fat: 7g
- Fiber: 3g

Serves

- 4 pancakes

Cooking Time

- 20 minutes

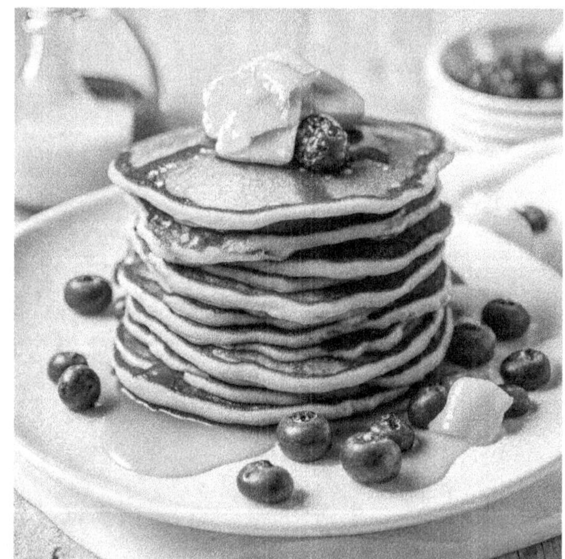

12. Egg Muffins

Ingredients

- 6 large eggs
- 1/4 cup lactose-free milk or almond milk
- 1/2 cup spinach, chopped
- 1/2 red bell pepper, diced
- 1/4 cup lactose-free cheese, shredded (optional)
- 1 teaspoon dried oregano

Instructions

1. Preheat your oven to 375°F (190°C) and grease a muffin tin with a little oil.
2. In a large bowl, whisk together the eggs and milk.
3. Stir in the chopped spinach, diced bell pepper, shredded cheese (if using), and oregano.
4. Pour the egg mixture into the muffin tin, filling each cup about 3/4 full.
5. Bake for 20-25 minutes until the muffins are set and golden brown.
6. Let cool for a few minutes before removing from the tin. Serve warm or store in the refrigerator for up to 4 days.

Nutrition Info per Serving

- Calories: 80
- Protein: 6g
- Carbohydrates: 2g
- Fat: 5g
- Fiber: 1g

Serves

- 6 muffins

Cooking Time

- 30 minutes

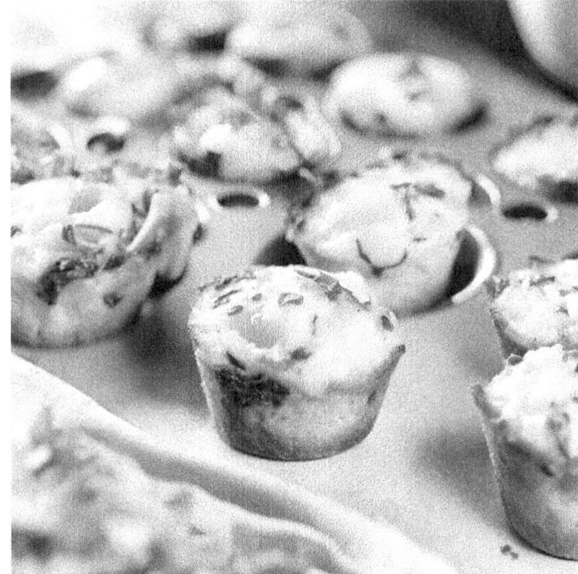

13. Savory Porridge

Ingredients

- 1 cup rolled oats (gluten-free)
- 2 cups water or lactose-free milk
- 1/2 cup spinach, chopped
- 1/2 avocado, sliced
- 1 tablespoon chia seeds
- 1 teaspoon turmeric
- 1/4 teaspoon cumin
- 1/4 cup cherry tomatoes, halved

Instructions

1. In a medium saucepan, bring water or milk to a boil. Add rolled oats and reduce heat to a simmer.
2. Cook for 5 minutes, stirring occasionally, until oats are soft and creamy.
3. Stir in chopped spinach, chia seeds, turmeric, and cumin. Cook for another 2 minutes until spinach is wilted.
4. Remove from heat and let sit for a few minutes to thicken.
5. Serve topped with sliced avocado and cherry tomatoes.

Nutrition Info per Serving

- Calories: 220
- Protein: 7g
- Carbohydrates: 30g
- Fat: 9g
- Fiber: 6g

Serves

- 2

Cooking Time

- 10 minutes

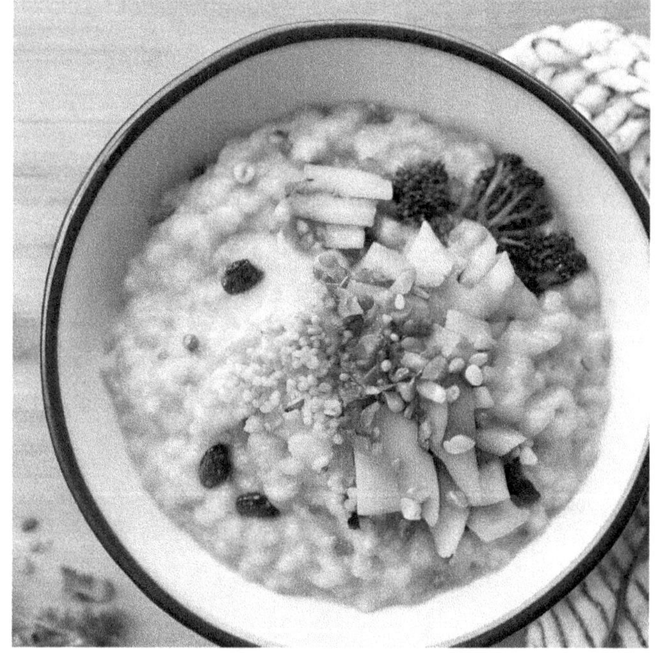

14. Pumpkin Pancakes

Ingredients

- 1 cup almond flour
- 1/2 cup pumpkin puree
- 2 large eggs
- 1/4 cup lactose-free milk or almond milk
- 1 tablespoon maple syrup
- 1 teaspoon cinnamon
- 1/2 teaspoon baking powder

Instructions

1. In a large bowl, mix together almond flour, pumpkin puree, eggs, milk, maple syrup, cinnamon, and baking powder until smooth.
2. Heat a non-stick skillet over medium heat and lightly grease with a little oil.
3. Pour 1/4 cup of batter onto the skillet for each pancake. Cook until bubbles form on the surface, then flip and cook until golden brown.
4. Serve warm with additional maple syrup and a sprinkle of cinnamon.

Nutrition Info per Serving

- Calories: 180
- Protein: 6g
- Carbohydrates: 12g
- Fat: 13g
- Fiber: 3g

Serves

- 4 pancakes

Cooking Time

- 20 minutes

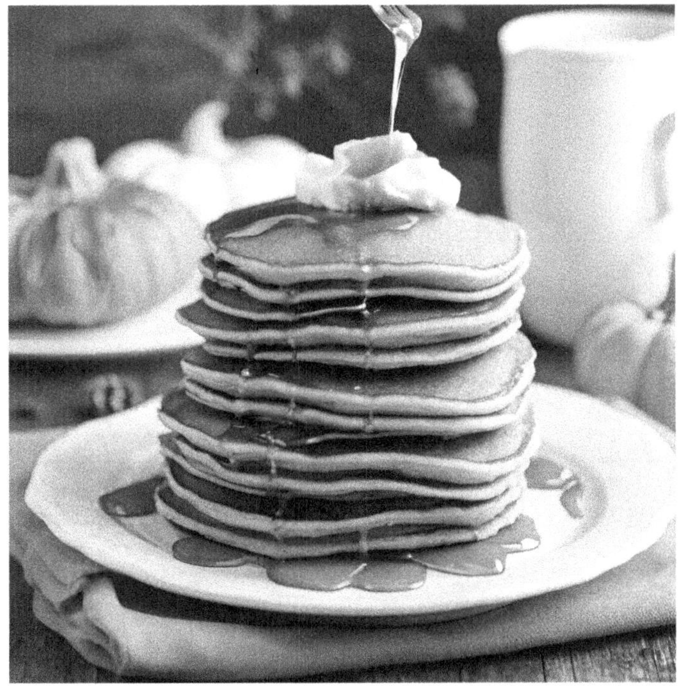

15. Smoked Salmon and Avocado Toast

Ingredients

- 4 slices gluten-free sourdough bread
- 1 avocado, mashed
- 1 teaspoon lemon juice
- 4 ounces smoked salmon
- 1 teaspoon capers
- 1 teaspoon dill, chopped

Instructions

1. Toast the sourdough bread slices until golden brown.
2. In a bowl, mash the avocado and mix with lemon juice.
3. Spread the avocado mixture evenly over each slice of toast.
4. Top each toast with smoked salmon, capers, and chopped dill.
5. Serve immediately.

Nutrition Info per Serving

- Calories: 250
- Protein: 12g
- Carbohydrates: 20g
- Fat: 14g
- Fiber: 5g

Serves

- 2

Cooking Time

- 10 minutes

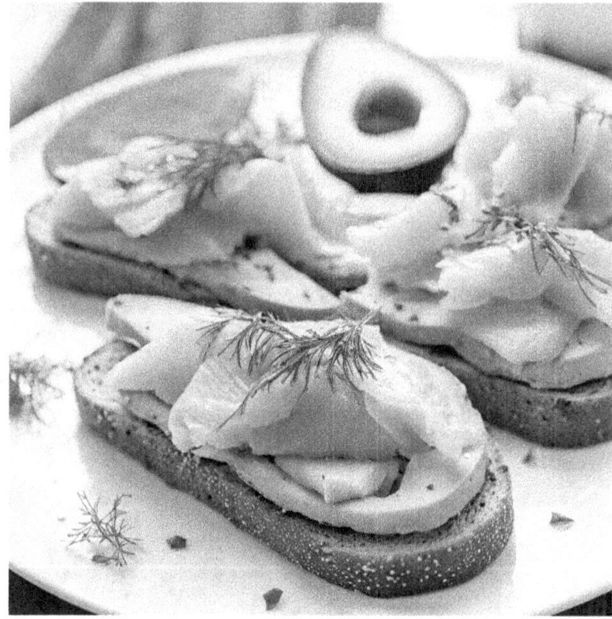

16. Raspberry Smoothie Bowl

Ingredients

- 1 cup frozen raspberries
- 1 banana, sliced
- 1/2 cup lactose-free yogurt or coconut yogurt
- 1/2 cup almond milk
- 1 tablespoon chia seeds
- 1 tablespoon almond butter
- 1/4 cup granola (gluten-free)

Instructions

1. In a blender, combine frozen raspberries, banana, yogurt, almond milk, chia seeds, and almond butter. Blend until smooth.
2. Pour the smoothie into a bowl.
3. Top with granola and additional raspberries if desired.
4. Serve immediately.

Nutrition Info per Serving

- Calories: 300
- Protein: 7g
- Carbohydrates: 45g
- Fat: 12g
- Fiber: 10g

Serves

- 2

Cooking Time

- 10 minutes

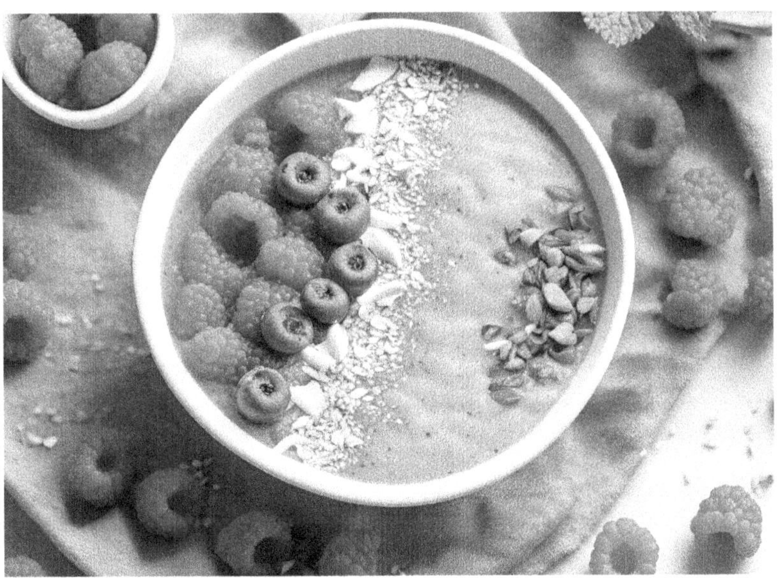

17. Strawberry Oat Bars

Ingredients

- 2 cups gluten-free oats
- 1/2 cup almond flour
- 1/4 cup coconut oil, melted
- 1/4 cup maple syrup
- 1 teaspoon vanilla extract
- 1 cup strawberries, chopped

Instructions

1. Preheat the oven to 350°F (175°C) and line an 8x8 inch baking pan with parchment paper.
2. In a large bowl, mix together oats, almond flour, coconut oil, maple syrup, and vanilla extract until well combined.
3. Press half of the mixture into the bottom of the prepared baking pan.
4. Spread the chopped strawberries evenly over the oat mixture.
5. Sprinkle the remaining oat mixture over the strawberries, pressing gently.
6. Bake for 25-30 minutes, until the top is golden brown.
7. Allow to cool completely before cutting into bars.

Nutrition Info per Serving

- Calories: 180
- Protein: 3g
- Carbohydrates: 24g
- Fat: 8g
- Fiber: 4g

Serves

- 8 bars

Cooking Time

- 35 minutes

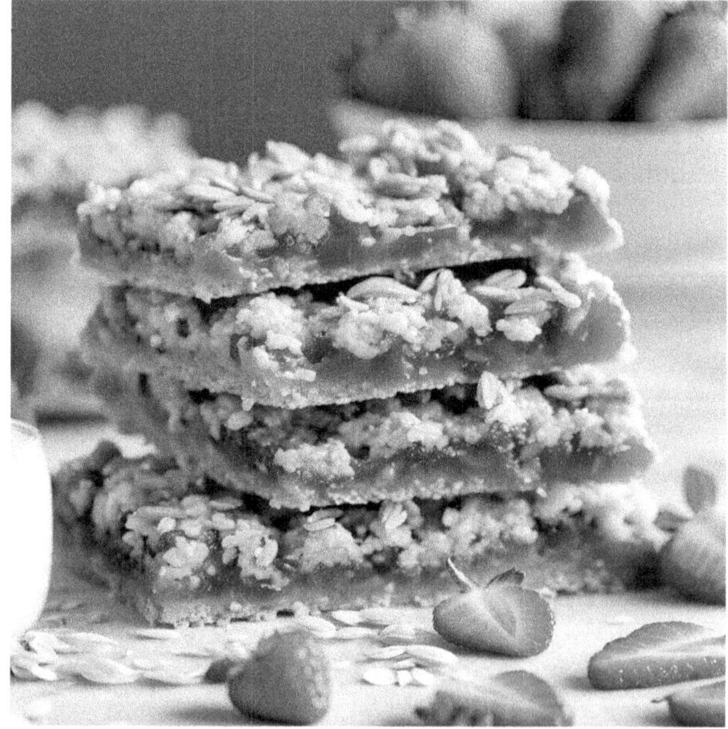

18. Protein Shake

Ingredients

- 1 cup lactose-free milk or almond milk
- 1 scoop low FODMAP protein powder (such as whey isolate or pea protein)
- 1/2 banana, sliced
- 1 tablespoon almond butter
- 1 teaspoon chia seeds
- 1/2 teaspoon vanilla extract
- 4-5 ice cubes

Instructions

1. Place all ingredients in a blender.
2. Blend on high speed until smooth and creamy.
3. Pour into a glass and serve immediately.

Nutrition Info per Serving

- Calories: 280
- Protein: 20g
- Carbohydrates: 24g
- Fat: 12g
- Fiber: 6g

Serves

- 1

Cooking Time

- 5 minutes

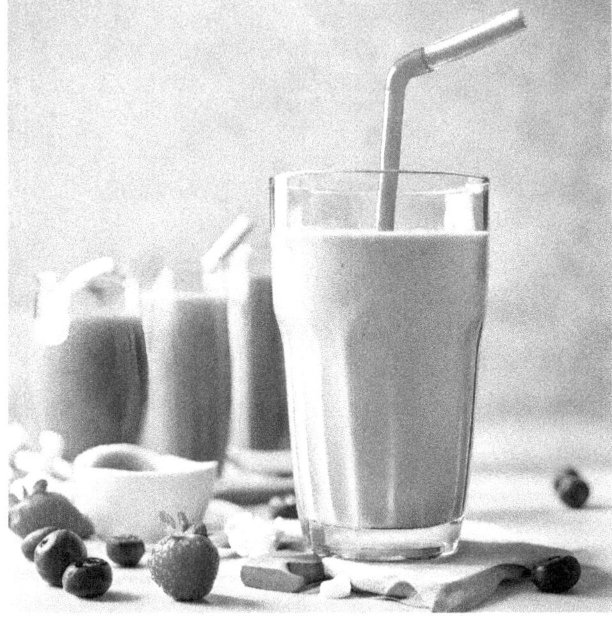

19. Almond Porridge

Ingredients

- 1/2 cup almond flour
- 1 cup lactose-free milk or almond milk
- 1 tablespoon chia seeds
- 1 tablespoon maple syrup
- 1/2 teaspoon cinnamon
- 1/4 cup blueberries

Instructions

1. In a small saucepan, combine almond flour, milk, chia seeds, maple syrup, and cinnamon.
2. Cook over medium heat, stirring constantly, until the mixture thickens, about 5-7 minutes.
3. Remove from heat and let sit for a few minutes to thicken further.
4. Serve topped with blueberries.

Nutrition Info per Serving

- Calories: 300
- Protein: 10g
- Carbohydrates: 28g
- Fat: 18g
- Fiber: 8g

Serves

- 1

Cooking Time

- 10 minutes

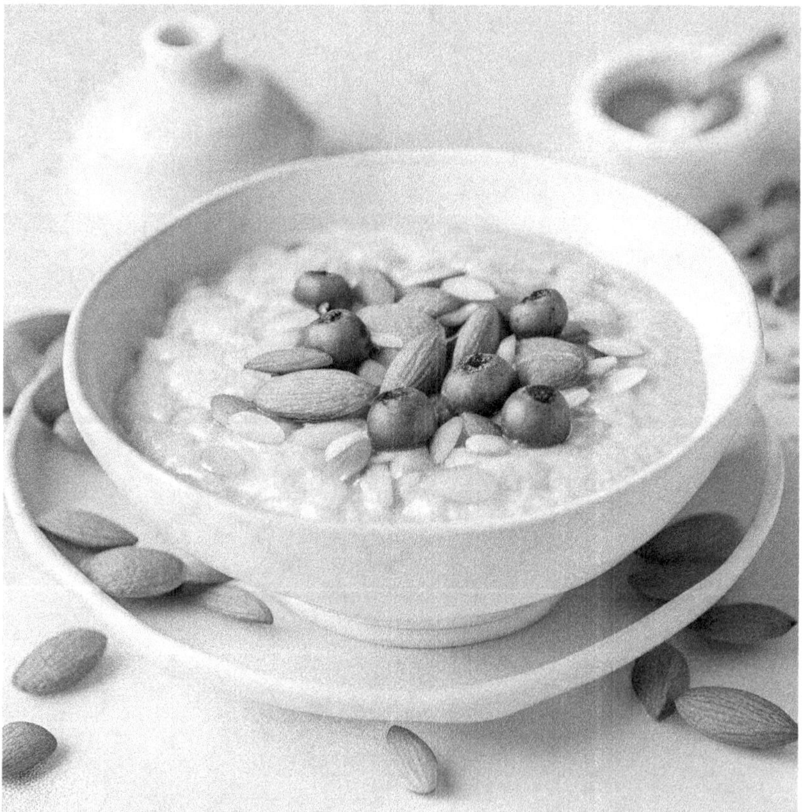

20. Bacon Lettuce Tomato (BLT) Sandwich

Ingredients

- 4 slices gluten-free bread
- 4 slices cooked bacon (nitrate-free)
- 4 lettuce leaves
- 1 tomato, sliced
- 2 tablespoons mayonnaise (lactose-free)
- 1 teaspoon Dijon mustard

Instructions

1. Toast the gluten-free bread slices until golden brown.
2. In a small bowl, mix the mayonnaise and Dijon mustard.
3. Spread the mayonnaise mixture evenly over the toasted bread slices.
4. Layer the lettuce, tomato slices, and bacon on two slices of the bread.
5. Top with the remaining slices of bread to make sandwiches.
6. Cut in half and serve immediately.

Nutrition Info per Serving

- Calories: 350
- Protein: 15g
- Carbohydrates: 28g
- Fat: 20g
- Fiber: 4g

Serves

- 2 sandwiches

Cooking Time

- 15 minutes

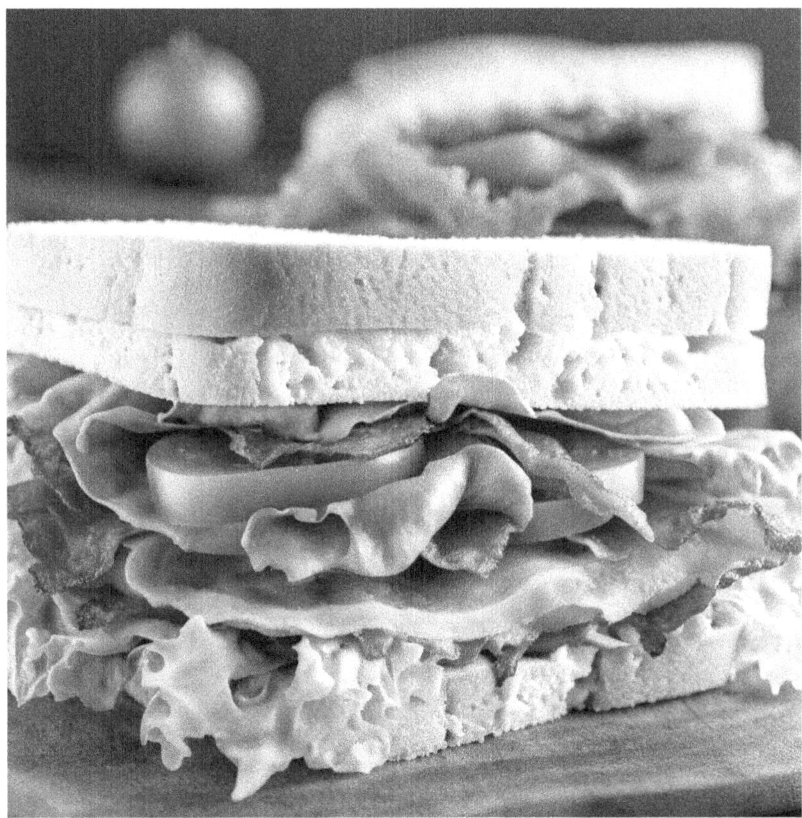

21. Pineapple and Cucumber Salad

Ingredients

- 1 cup fresh pineapple, diced
- 1 cucumber, sliced
- 1 tablespoon lime juice
- 1 tablespoon fresh mint, chopped
- 1 teaspoon olive oil

Instructions

1. In a large bowl, combine diced pineapple and sliced cucumber.
2. Drizzle with lime juice and olive oil.
3. Toss to combine.
4. Garnish with chopped fresh mint before serving.

Nutrition Info per Serving

- Calories: 80
- Protein: 1g
- Carbohydrates: 15g
- Fat: 2g
- Fiber: 2g

Serves

- 2

Cooking Time

- 10 minutes

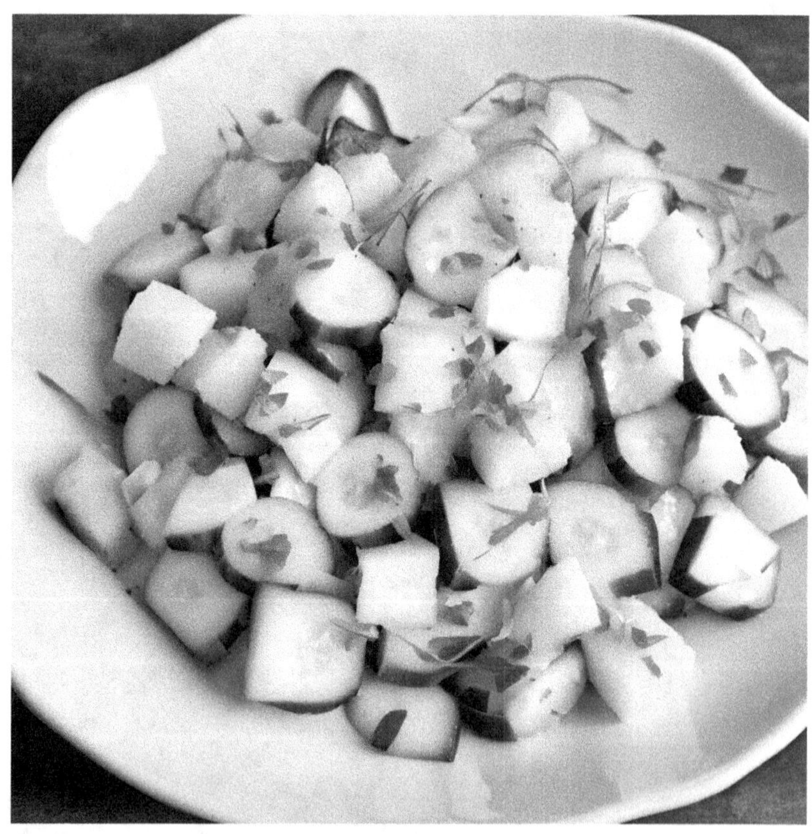

Beef and Pork Recipes

1. Beef Carpaccio

Ingredients

- 8 ounces beef tenderloin, thinly sliced
- 2 tablespoons olive oil
- 1 tablespoon lemon juice
- 1 cup arugula
- 2 tablespoons shaved Parmesan cheese
- 1 tablespoon capers, drained
- 1 teaspoon Dijon mustard

Instructions

1. Freeze the beef tenderloin for 1 hour to make it easier to slice thinly.
2. Using a sharp knife, slice the beef as thinly as possible and arrange the slices on a large plate.
3. In a small bowl, whisk together olive oil, lemon juice, and Dijon mustard.
4. Drizzle the dressing over the beef slices.
5. Top with arugula, shaved Parmesan, and capers.
6. Serve immediately.

Nutrition Info per Serving

- Calories: 210
- Protein: 19g
- Carbohydrates: 3g
- Fat: 14g
- Fiber: 1g

Serves

- 2

Cooking Time

- 10 minutes (plus 1 hour freezing time)

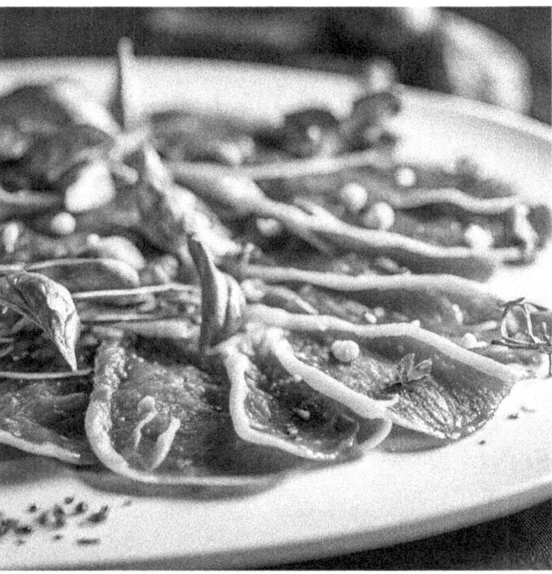

2. Pork Pad Thai

Ingredients

- 8 ounces rice noodles
- 1 tablespoon olive oil
- 1 pound pork tenderloin, thinly sliced
- 1/2 cup carrots, julienned
- 1/2 cup bell peppers, thinly sliced
- 2 eggs, beaten
- 1/4 cup peanuts, chopped
- 1/4 cup green onions, chopped
- 1/4 cup fresh cilantro, chopped
- 3 tablespoons fish sauce
- 2 tablespoons lime juice
- 1 tablespoon brown sugar
- 1 teaspoon chili flakes

Instructions

1. Cook the rice noodles according to package instructions, then drain and set aside.
2. In a large skillet or wok, heat olive oil over medium-high heat.
3. Add the pork slices and cook until browned, about 5-7 minutes.
4. Add the carrots and bell peppers, and cook for another 3-4 minutes.
5. Push the pork and vegetables to one side of the skillet and add the beaten eggs to the empty side. Scramble the eggs until cooked, then mix them with the pork and vegetables.
6. Add the cooked noodles to the skillet and toss to combine.
7. In a small bowl, mix fish sauce, lime juice, brown sugar, and chili flakes. Pour over the noodle mixture and toss to coat evenly.
8. Serve topped with chopped peanuts, green onions, and fresh cilantro.

Nutrition Info per Serving

- Calories: 450
- Protein: 25g
- Carbohydrates: 55g
- Fat: 15g
- Fiber: 4g

Serves

- 4

Cooking Time

- 25 minutes

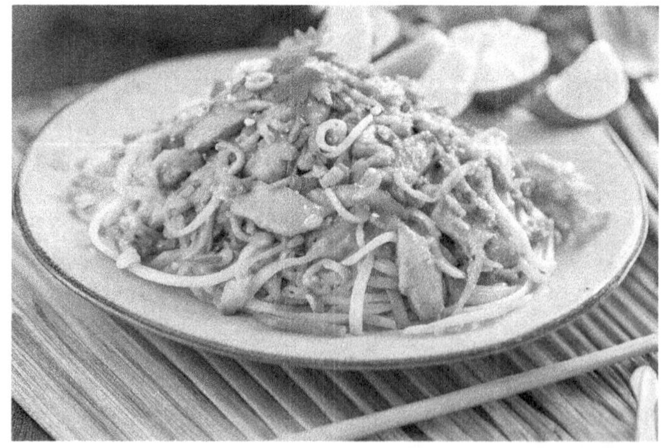

3. Beef Liver

Ingredients

- 1 pound beef liver, thinly sliced
- 1/2 cup gluten-free flour
- 2 tablespoons olive oil
- 1 onion, thinly sliced
- 1/4 cup balsamic vinegar
- 1/4 cup fresh parsley, chopped

Instructions

1. Dredge the beef liver slices in gluten-free flour.
2. In a large skillet, heat olive oil over medium-high heat.
3. Add the liver slices and cook for 3-4 minutes on each side until browned and cooked through.
4. Remove the liver from the skillet and set aside.
5. In the same skillet, add the sliced onion and cook for 5-7 minutes until caramelized.
6. Add balsamic vinegar to the skillet and stir to deglaze, scraping up any browned bits.
7. Return the liver to the skillet and cook for an additional 2 minutes.
8. Garnish with fresh parsley before serving.

Nutrition Info per Serving

- Calories: 250
- Protein: 28g
- Carbohydrates: 10g
- Fat: 10g
- Fiber: 2g

Serves

- 4

Cooking Time

- 20 minutes

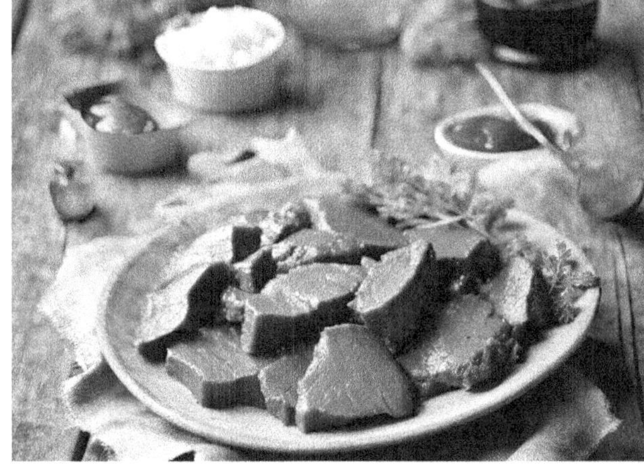

4. Pork Fajitas
Ingredients

- 1 pound pork loin, thinly sliced
- 2 tablespoons olive oil
- 1 red bell pepper, thinly sliced
- 1 green bell pepper, thinly sliced
- 1 onion, thinly sliced
- 1 teaspoon cumin
- 1 teaspoon paprika
- 8 gluten-free tortillas
- 1/2 cup lactose-free sour cream (optional)
- 1/2 cup fresh cilantro, chopped

Instructions

1. In a large skillet, heat olive oil over medium-high heat.
2. Add the sliced pork and cook until browned, about 5-7 minutes.
3. Add the bell peppers and onion to the skillet and cook for another 5-7 minutes until the vegetables are tender.
4. Sprinkle cumin and paprika over the pork and vegetables, and toss to coat evenly.
5. Warm the tortillas according to package instructions.
6. Serve the pork and vegetable mixture in the tortillas, topped with lactose-free sour cream (if using) and fresh cilantro.

Nutrition Info per Serving

- Calories: 350
- Protein: 20g
- Carbohydrates: 40g
- Fat: 12g
- Fiber: 5g

Serves

- 4

Cooking Time

- 20 minutes

5. Beef Shepherd's Pie

Ingredients

- 1 pound ground beef
- 1 onion, diced
- 1 cup carrots, diced
- 1 cup peas (frozen or fresh)
- 1 cup beef broth
- 2 tablespoons tomato paste
- 4 cups mashed potatoes (made with lactose-free milk and butter)
- 1 tablespoon olive oil

Instructions

1. Preheat your oven to 375°F (190°C).
2. In a large skillet, heat olive oil over medium heat. Add the diced onion and cook until softened, about 5 minutes.
3. Add the ground beef to the skillet and cook until browned, breaking it up with a spoon.
4. Stir in the carrots and cook for another 5 minutes.
5. Add the tomato paste and beef broth, stirring to combine. Simmer for 10 minutes until the carrots are tender.
6. Stir in the peas and cook for an additional 2 minutes.
7. Transfer the beef mixture to a baking dish and spread it out evenly.
8. Top with the mashed potatoes, spreading them out to cover the beef mixture completely.
9. Bake for 25-30 minutes until the top is golden brown.
10. Let cool for a few minutes before serving.

Nutrition Info per Serving

- Calories: 400
- Protein: 22g
- Carbohydrates: 40g
- Fat: 18g
- Fiber: 6g

Serves

- 4

Cooking Time

- 45 minutes

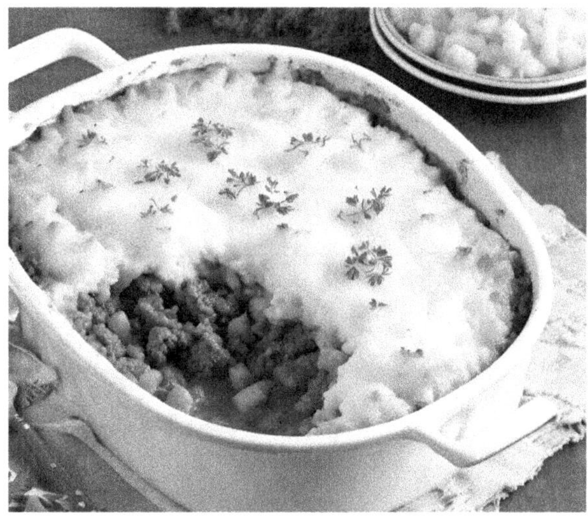

6. Pork and Herb Sausages

Ingredients

- 1 pound ground pork
- 1 tablespoon fresh sage, finely chopped
- 1 tablespoon fresh rosemary, finely chopped
- 1 tablespoon fresh thyme, finely chopped
- 1 teaspoon garlic-infused oil
- 1/2 teaspoon smoked paprika
- 1 tablespoon olive oil (for cooking)

Instructions

1. In a large bowl, combine ground pork, sage, rosemary, thyme, garlic-infused oil, and smoked paprika. Mix until well combined.
2. Divide the mixture into 8 equal portions and shape into sausage links or patties.
3. Heat olive oil in a large skillet over medium heat.
4. Add the sausages and cook for 4-5 minutes on each side, until browned and cooked through.
5. Serve immediately.

Nutrition Info per Serving

- Calories: 180
- Protein: 15g
- Carbohydrates: 1g
- Fat: 13g
- Fiber: 0g

Serves

- 4 (2 sausages each)

Cooking Time

- 20 minutes

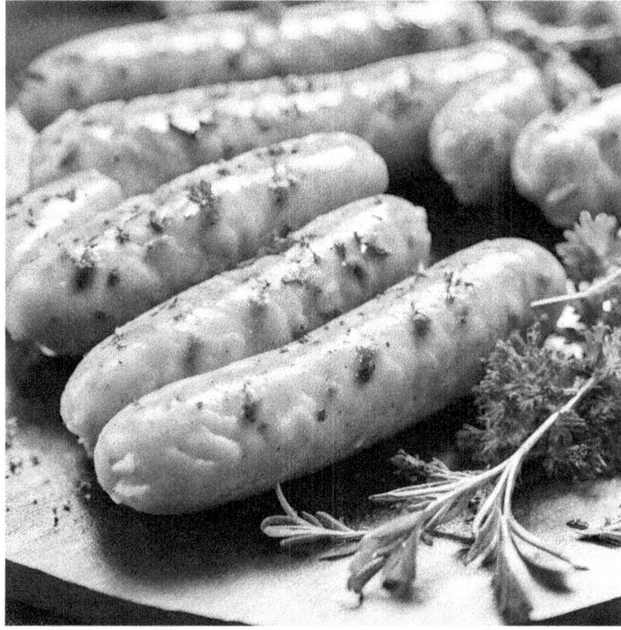

7. Beef Ragout

Ingredients

- 1 pound beef stew meat, cubed
- 2 tablespoons olive oil
- 1 onion, diced
- 2 carrots, diced
- 1 cup diced tomatoes (canned, no added salt)
- 2 cups beef broth
- 1 teaspoon dried thyme
- 1 teaspoon dried oregano
- 1/2 cup red wine (optional)
- 1 tablespoon fresh parsley, chopped (for garnish)

Instructions

1. In a large pot, heat olive oil over medium-high heat.
2. Add beef stew meat and cook until browned on all sides, about 5-7 minutes.
3. Remove the beef from the pot and set aside.
4. In the same pot, add diced onion and carrots. Cook until the vegetables are softened, about 5 minutes.
5. Return the beef to the pot. Add diced tomatoes, beef broth, thyme, oregano, and red wine (if using).
6. Bring the mixture to a boil, then reduce the heat to low. Cover and simmer for 1.5 to 2 hours, until the beef is tender.
7. Garnish with fresh parsley before serving.

Nutrition Info per Serving

- Calories: 280
- Protein: 25g
- Carbohydrates: 10g
- Fat: 15g
- Fiber: 3g

Serves

- 4

Cooking Time

- 2 hours 15 minutes

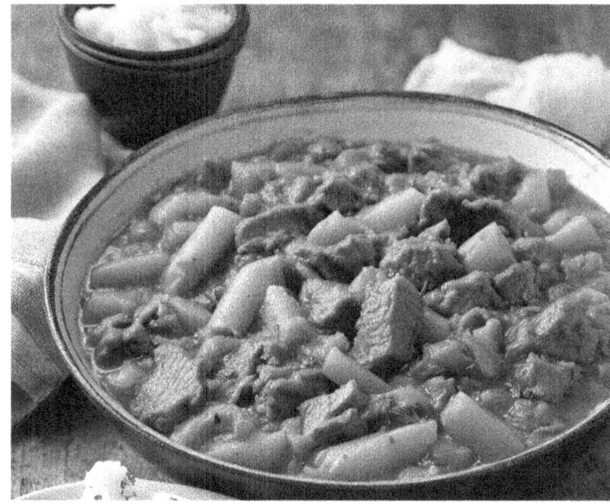

8. Pork Schnitzel

Ingredients

- 4 boneless pork chops
- 1/2 cup gluten-free breadcrumbs
- 1/4 cup gluten-free flour
- 2 large eggs, beaten
- 2 tablespoons olive oil
- 1 tablespoon lemon juice
- 1 tablespoon fresh parsley, chopped (for garnish)

Instructions

1. Place each pork chop between two sheets of plastic wrap and pound with a meat mallet until about 1/4-inch thick.
2. Set up a breading station with three shallow dishes: one with gluten-free flour, one with beaten eggs, and one with gluten-free breadcrumbs.
3. Dredge each pork chop in the flour, dip in the eggs, and coat with breadcrumbs.
4. In a large skillet, heat olive oil over medium-high heat.
5. Add the breaded pork chops and cook for 3-4 minutes on each side, until golden brown and cooked through.
6. Remove from heat and drizzle with lemon juice. Garnish with fresh parsley before serving.

Nutrition Info per Serving

- Calories: 350
- Protein: 30g
- Carbohydrates: 20g
- Fat: 15g
- Fiber: 2g

Serves

- 4

Cooking Time

- 20 minutes

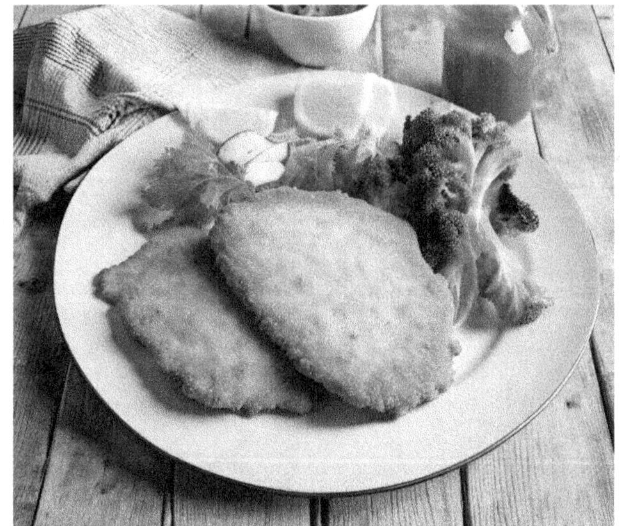

9. Beef Jerky

Ingredients

- 1 pound beef sirloin, thinly sliced
- 1/4 cup tamari (gluten-free soy sauce)
- 1 tablespoon Worcestershire sauce (gluten-free)
- 1 tablespoon maple syrup
- 1 teaspoon garlic-infused oil
- 1 teaspoon smoked paprika

Instructions

1. In a large bowl, combine tamari, Worcestershire sauce, maple syrup, garlic-infused oil, and smoked paprika.
2. Add the beef slices to the marinade, ensuring each piece is well-coated. Cover and refrigerate for at least 4 hours, preferably overnight.
3. Preheat the oven to 175°F (80°C). Line a baking sheet with parchment paper and place a wire rack on top.
4. Arrange the marinated beef slices on the wire rack in a single layer.
5. Bake for 3-4 hours, until the beef is dry and slightly pliable.
6. Let cool completely before storing in an airtight container.

Nutrition Info per Serving

- Calories: 150
- Protein: 20g
- Carbohydrates: 5g
- Fat: 5g
- Fiber: 0g

Serves

- 8

Cooking Time

- 4 hours 15 minutes (plus marinating time)

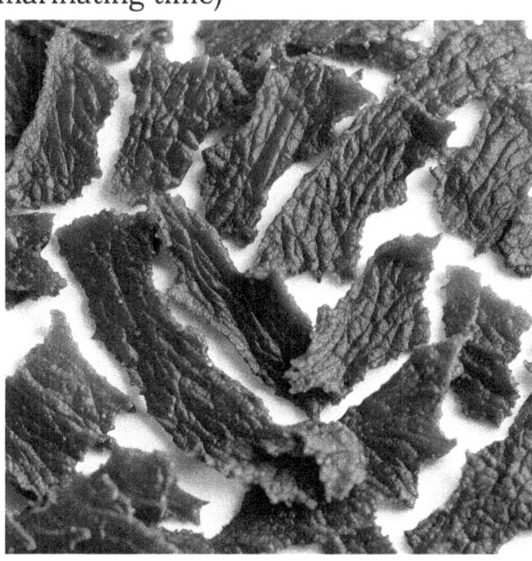

10. Spareribs

Ingredients

- 2 pounds pork spareribs
- 1/4 cup low-sodium tamari (gluten-free soy sauce)
- 1/4 cup maple syrup
- 1/4 cup apple cider vinegar
- 1 tablespoon garlic-infused oil
- 1 teaspoon smoked paprika
- 1 teaspoon dried thyme

Instructions

1. Preheat your oven to 300°F (150°C).
2. In a small bowl, mix together tamari, maple syrup, apple cider vinegar, garlic-infused oil, smoked paprika, and thyme.
3. Place the spareribs in a baking dish and pour the marinade over them, ensuring they are well-coated.
4. Cover the baking dish with aluminum foil and bake for 2.5 to 3 hours, until the meat is tender and easily pulls away from the bone.
5. Remove the foil and increase the oven temperature to 400°F (200°C). Bake for an additional 15 minutes to allow the ribs to caramelize.
6. Let the ribs rest for 10 minutes before serving.

Nutrition Info per Serving

- Calories: 400
- Protein: 28g
- Carbohydrates: 10g
- Fat: 28g
- Fiber: 1g

Serves

- 4

Cooking Time

- 3 hours 30 minutes

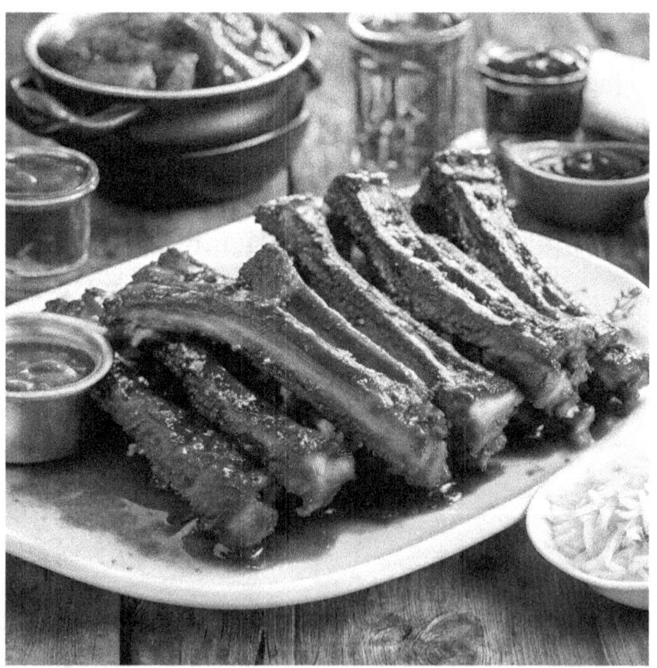

11. Pork Goulash

Ingredients

- 1 pound pork shoulder, cubed
- 2 tablespoons olive oil
- 1 onion, diced
- 2 red bell peppers, diced
- 1 cup diced tomatoes (canned, no added salt)
- 2 cups chicken broth
- 1 tablespoon paprika
- 1 teaspoon caraway seeds
- 1 tablespoon fresh parsley, chopped (for garnish)

Instructions

1. In a large pot, heat olive oil over medium-high heat.
2. Add the diced onion and cook until softened, about 5 minutes.
3. Add the cubed pork shoulder and cook until browned on all sides, about 8-10 minutes.
4. Add the bell peppers, diced tomatoes, chicken broth, paprika, and caraway seeds. Stir to combine.
5. Bring to a boil, then reduce heat to low and simmer for 1.5 to 2 hours, until the pork is tender.
6. Garnish with fresh parsley before serving.

Nutrition Info per Serving

- Calories: 320
- Protein: 28g
- Carbohydrates: 15g
- Fat: 16g
- Fiber: 4g

Serves

- 4

Cooking Time

- 2 hours 20 minutes

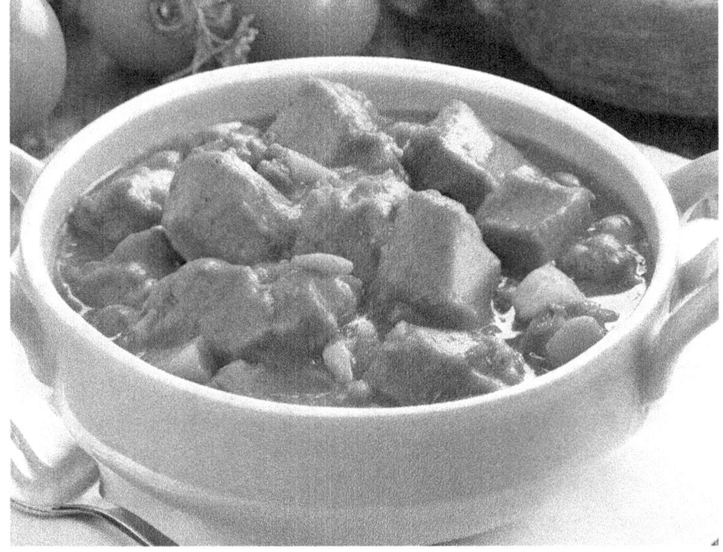

12. Beef Brisket

Ingredients

- 2 pounds beef brisket
- 1/4 cup low-sodium tamari (gluten-free soy sauce)
- 1/4 cup apple cider vinegar
- 1/4 cup maple syrup
- 1 tablespoon garlic-infused oil
- 1 teaspoon smoked paprika
- 1 teaspoon dried thyme

Instructions

1. Preheat your oven to 300°F (150°C).
2. In a small bowl, mix together tamari, apple cider vinegar, maple syrup, garlic-infused oil, smoked paprika, and thyme.
3. Place the beef brisket in a baking dish and pour the marinade over it, ensuring it is well-coated.
4. Cover the baking dish with aluminum foil and bake for 3 to 3.5 hours, until the meat is tender and easily pulls apart.
5. Remove the foil and increase the oven temperature to 400°F (200°C). Bake for an additional 15 minutes to allow the brisket to caramelize.
6. Let the brisket rest for 10 minutes before slicing and serving.

Nutrition Info per Serving

- Calories: 380
- Protein: 30g
- Carbohydrates: 10g
- Fat: 24g
- Fiber: 1g

Serves

- 4

Cooking Time

- 3 hours 45 minutes

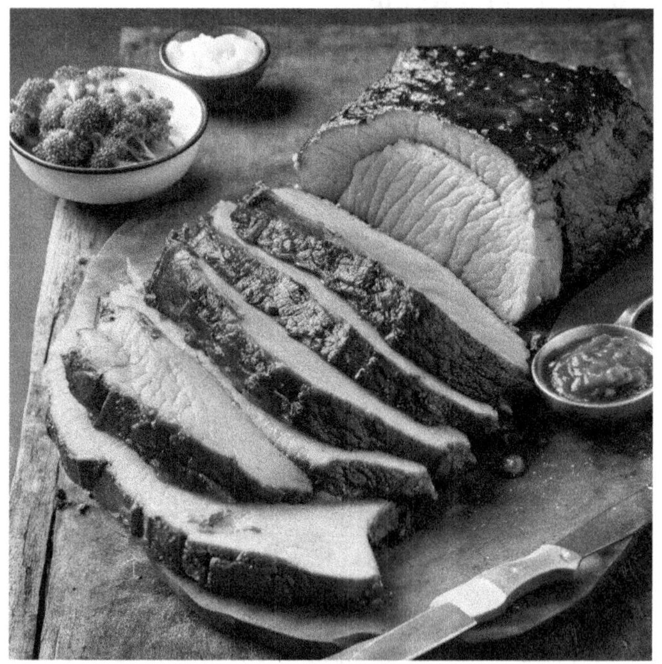

13. Pork Stew
Ingredients
- 1 pound pork shoulder, cubed
- 2 tablespoons olive oil
- 1 onion, diced
- 2 carrots, diced
- 2 potatoes, cubed
- 1 cup diced tomatoes (canned, no added salt)
- 2 cups chicken broth
- 1 teaspoon dried thyme
- 1 teaspoon paprika
- 1 bay leaf

Instructions
1. In a large pot, heat olive oil over medium-high heat.
2. Add the diced onion and cook until softened, about 5 minutes.
3. Add the cubed pork shoulder and cook until browned on all sides, about 8-10 minutes.
4. Add the carrots, potatoes, diced tomatoes, chicken broth, thyme, paprika, and bay leaf. Stir to combine.
5. Bring to a boil, then reduce heat to low and simmer for 1.5 to 2 hours, until the pork and vegetables are tender.
6. Remove the bay leaf before serving.

Nutrition Info per Serving
- Calories: 320
- Protein: 25g
- Carbohydrates: 25g
- Fat: 12g
- Fiber: 4g

Serves
- 4

Cooking Time
- 2 hours 20 minutes

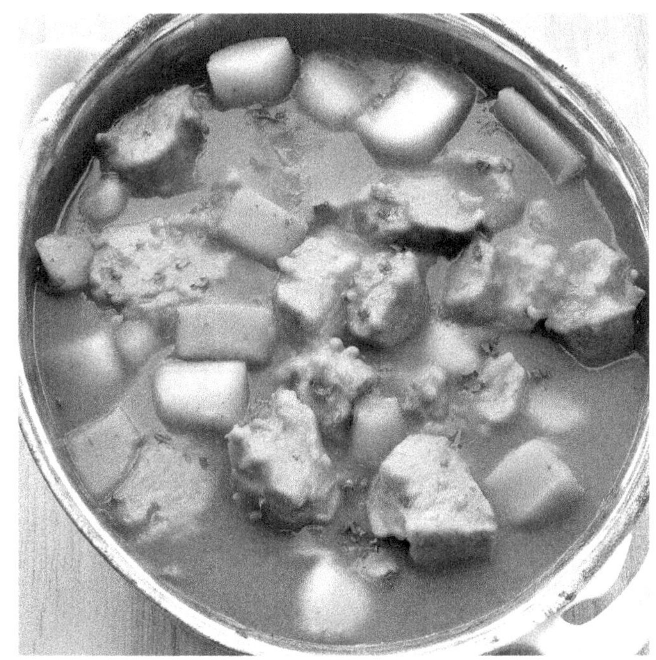

14. Meatloaf

Ingredients

- 1 pound ground beef
- 1/2 cup gluten-free breadcrumbs
- 1/4 cup lactose-free milk
- 1 egg
- 1 onion, finely diced
- 1 tablespoon Worcestershire sauce (gluten-free)
- 1 tablespoon tomato paste
- 1 teaspoon dried thyme

Instructions

1. Preheat your oven to 350°F (175°C).
2. In a large bowl, combine ground beef, gluten-free breadcrumbs, milk, egg, diced onion, Worcestershire sauce, tomato paste, and thyme. Mix until well combined.
3. Transfer the mixture to a loaf pan and shape it into a loaf.
4. Bake for 1 hour, until the meatloaf is cooked through and the internal temperature reaches 160°F (70°C).
5. Let the meatloaf rest for 10 minutes before slicing and serving.

Nutrition Info per Serving

- Calories: 300
- Protein: 25g
- Carbohydrates: 15g
- Fat: 16g
- Fiber: 2g

Serves

- 4

Cooking Time

- 1 hour 20 minutes

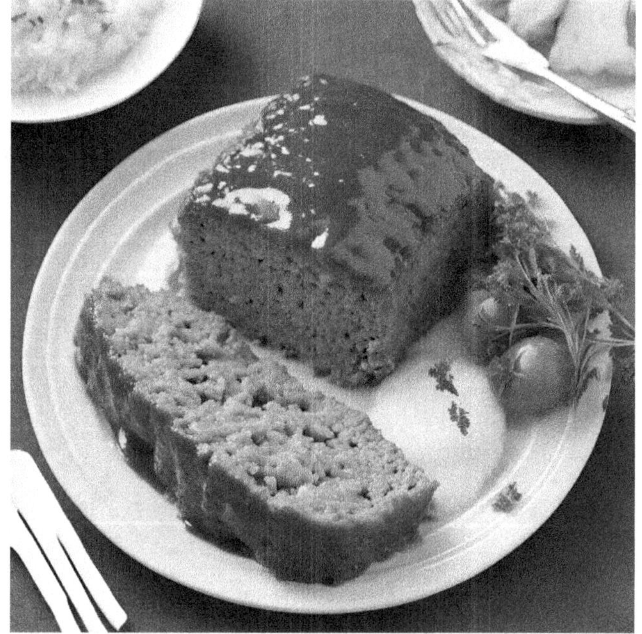

15. Pork Belly

Ingredients

- 2 pounds pork belly, skin scored
- 1/4 cup low-sodium tamari (gluten-free soy sauce)
- 1/4 cup apple cider vinegar
- 1/4 cup maple syrup
- 1 tablespoon garlic-infused oil
- 1 teaspoon Chinese five-spice powder

Instructions

1. Preheat your oven to 350°F (175°C).
2. In a small bowl, mix together tamari, apple cider vinegar, maple syrup, garlic-infused oil, and Chinese five-spice powder.
3. Place the pork belly in a baking dish and pour the marinade over it, ensuring it is well-coated.
4. Cover the baking dish with aluminum foil and bake for 2 hours.
5. Remove the foil and increase the oven temperature to 425°F (220°C). Bake for an additional 30-40 minutes, until the skin is crispy.
6. Let the pork belly rest for 10 minutes before slicing and serving.

Nutrition Info per Serving

- Calories: 450
- Protein: 20g
- Carbohydrates: 12g
- Fat: 36g
- Fiber: 0g

Serves

- 4

Cooking Time

- 2 hours 45 minutes

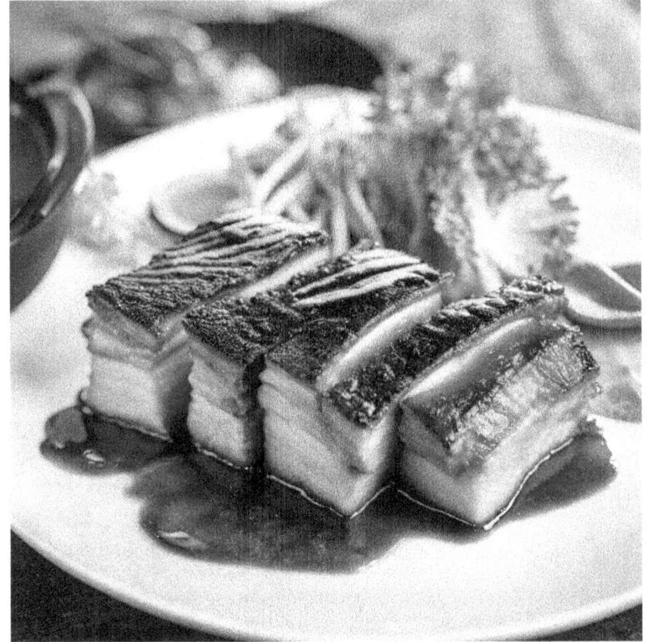

16. Beef Bourguignon

Ingredients

- 2 pounds beef chuck, cubed
- 4 strips bacon, diced
- 2 tablespoons olive oil
- 1 onion, diced
- 2 carrots, sliced
- 2 cups red wine (preferably Burgundy)
- 2 cups beef broth
- 1 tablespoon tomato paste
- 3 garlic-infused oil
- 1 teaspoon thyme
- 1 bay leaf
- 1 cup pearl onions (frozen, thawed)
- 1 cup mushrooms, sliced

Instructions

1. Preheat your oven to 350°F (175°C).
2. In a large Dutch oven, cook the bacon over medium heat until crisp. Remove bacon and set aside.
3. In the same pot, add olive oil and sear the beef cubes until browned on all sides. Remove and set aside.
4. Add the diced onion and carrots to the pot, and cook until softened, about 5 minutes.
5. Return the beef and bacon to the pot. Add the red wine, beef broth, tomato paste, garlic-infused oil, thyme, and bay leaf. Bring to a simmer.
6. Cover the pot and transfer to the oven. Cook for 2.5 to 3 hours, until the beef is tender.
7. In the last 30 minutes of cooking, add the pearl onions and mushrooms.
8. Serve hot, garnished with fresh thyme if desired.

Nutrition Info per Serving

- Calories: 400
- Protein: 32g
- Carbohydrates: 10g
- Fat: 20g
- Fiber: 2g

Serves

- 6

Cooking Time

- 3 hours 30 minutes

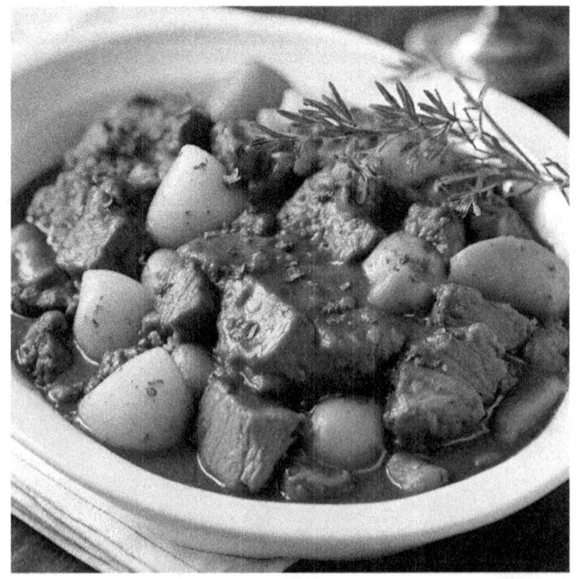

17. Italian Sausage

Ingredients

- 1 pound ground pork
- 1 teaspoon fennel seeds
- 1 teaspoon paprika
- 1/2 teaspoon red pepper flakes
- 1 teaspoon dried oregano
- 1 teaspoon dried basil
- 1 teaspoon garlic-infused oil

Instructions

1. In a large bowl, combine ground pork, fennel seeds, paprika, red pepper flakes, oregano, basil, and garlic-infused oil. Mix until well combined.
2. Divide the mixture into 8 equal portions and shape into sausage links or patties.
3. Heat a non-stick skillet over medium heat.
4. Cook the sausages for about 4-5 minutes on each side, until browned and cooked through.
5. Serve immediately.

Nutrition Info per Serving

- Calories: 180
- Protein: 14g
- Carbohydrates: 1g
- Fat: 13g
- Fiber: 0g

Serves

- 4 (2 sausages each)

Cooking Time

- 20 minutes

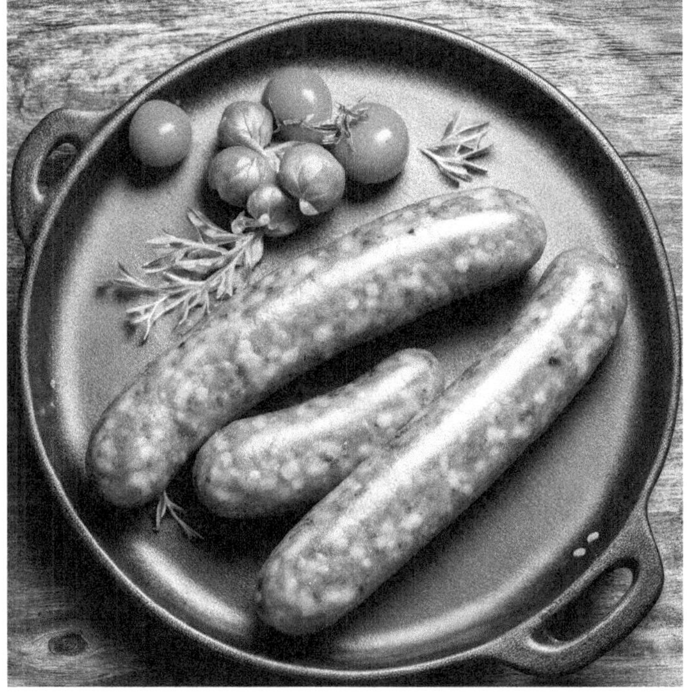

18. Pork Loin Roast

Ingredients

- 2 pounds pork loin roast
- 2 tablespoons olive oil
- 1 tablespoon garlic-infused oil
- 1 teaspoon dried rosemary
- 1 teaspoon dried thyme
- 1/2 cup chicken broth
- 1/2 cup apple cider vinegar

Instructions

1. Preheat your oven to 375°F (190°C).
2. In a small bowl, mix olive oil, garlic-infused oil, rosemary, and thyme.
3. Rub the mixture all over the pork loin.
4. Place the pork loin in a roasting pan. Pour chicken broth and apple cider vinegar into the bottom of the pan.
5. Roast in the preheated oven for 1 to 1.5 hours, until the internal temperature reaches 145°F (63°C).
6. Let the pork loin rest for 10 minutes before slicing and serving.

Nutrition Info per Serving

- Calories: 250
- Protein: 28g
- Carbohydrates: 2g
- Fat: 14g
- Fiber: 0g

Serves

- 6

Cooking Time

- 1 hour 30 minutes

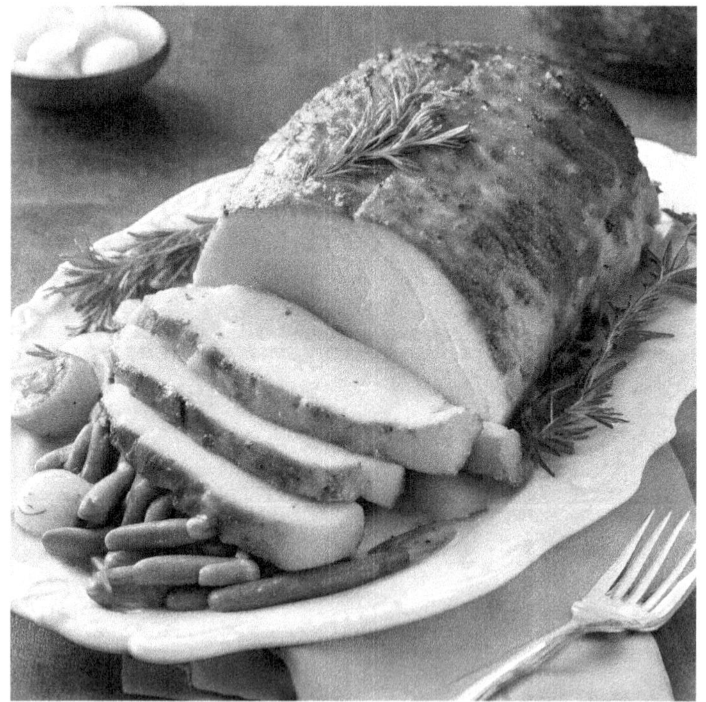

19. Bunless Beef Burgers

Ingredients

- 1 pound ground beef
- 1 tablespoon Worcestershire sauce (gluten-free)
- 1 teaspoon garlic-infused oil
- 1 teaspoon smoked paprika
- 1/2 teaspoon dried oregano
- 1 avocado, sliced
- 4 lettuce leaves
- 1 tomato, sliced

Instructions

1. In a large bowl, combine ground beef, Worcestershire sauce, garlic-infused oil, smoked paprika, and oregano. Mix until well combined.
2. Divide the mixture into 4 equal portions and shape into patties.
3. Heat a non-stick skillet or grill over medium-high heat.
4. Cook the patties for about 4-5 minutes on each side, until browned and cooked through.
5. Serve each patty on a lettuce leaf topped with avocado slices and tomato slices.

Nutrition Info per Serving

- Calories: 320
- Protein: 22g
- Carbohydrates: 4g
- Fat: 24g
- Fiber: 3g

Serves

- 4

Cooking Time

- 20 minutes

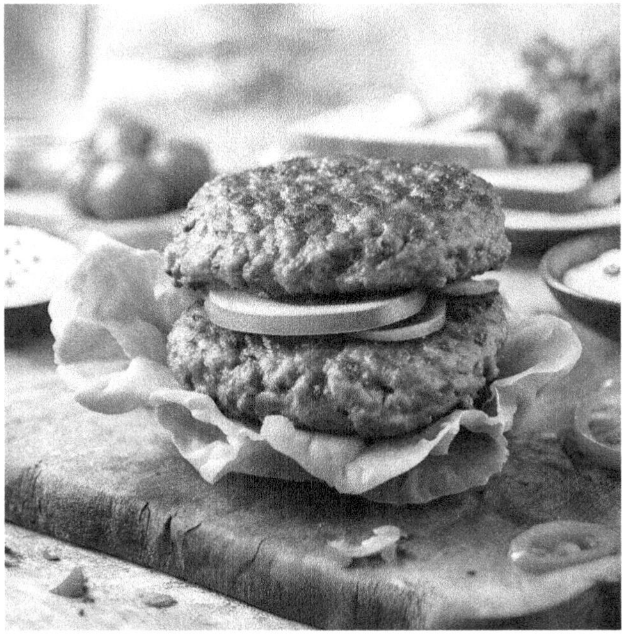

20. Pork and Chive Dumplings

Ingredients

- 1 pound ground pork
- 1/4 cup chives, finely chopped
- 1 tablespoon garlic-infused oil
- 1 tablespoon low-sodium tamari (gluten-free soy sauce)
- 1 teaspoon ginger, grated
- 24 gluten-free dumpling wrappers
- 2 tablespoons olive oil (for frying)
- 1/4 cup water (for steaming)

Instructions

1. In a large bowl, combine ground pork, chives, garlic-infused oil, tamari, and grated ginger. Mix until well combined.
2. Place a small spoonful of the pork mixture in the center of each dumpling wrapper.
3. Moisten the edges of the wrapper with water, fold in half, and press to seal.
4. Heat olive oil in a large non-stick skillet over medium-high heat.
5. Add the dumplings to the skillet and cook for 2-3 minutes until the bottoms are golden brown.
6. Carefully add 1/4 cup water to the skillet and cover. Steam for 5-6 minutes until the dumplings are cooked through.
7. Serve immediately.

Nutrition Info per Serving

- Calories: 250
- Protein: 18g
- Carbohydrates: 18g
- Fat: 12g
- Fiber: 2g

Serves

- 4

Cooking Time

- 30 minutes

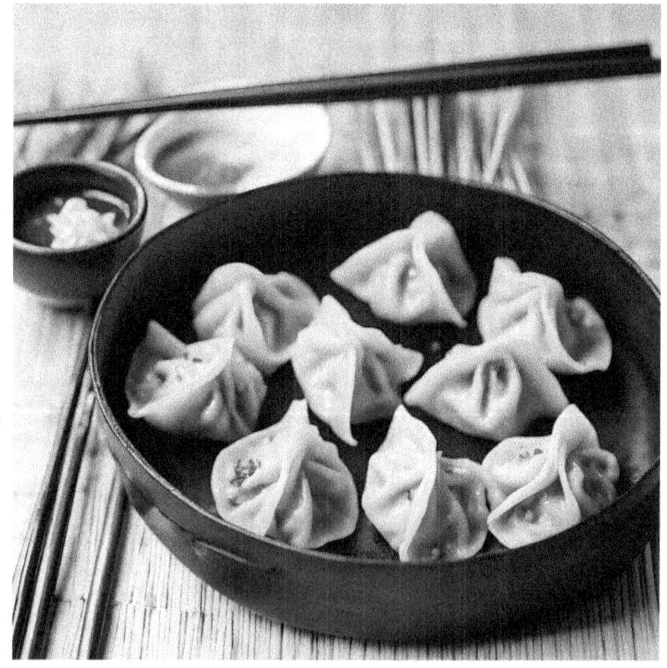

21. Pork Paillard

Ingredients

- 4 boneless pork chops
- 2 tablespoons olive oil
- 1 tablespoon lemon juice
- 1 teaspoon dried thyme
- 1/2 teaspoon smoked paprika
- 1/4 cup gluten-free flour

Instructions

1. Place each pork chop between two sheets of plastic wrap and pound with a meat mallet until about 1/4-inch thick.
2. In a small bowl, mix olive oil, lemon juice, thyme, and smoked paprika.
3. Brush the pork chops with the olive oil mixture, then dredge in gluten-free flour.
4. Heat a non-stick skillet over medium-high heat and add the pork chops.
5. Cook for 3-4 minutes on each side until golden brown and cooked through.
6. Serve immediately.

Nutrition Info per Serving

- Calories: 300
- Protein: 28g
- Carbohydrates: 10g
- Fat: 18g
- Fiber: 1g

Serves

- 4

Cooking Time

- 20 minutes

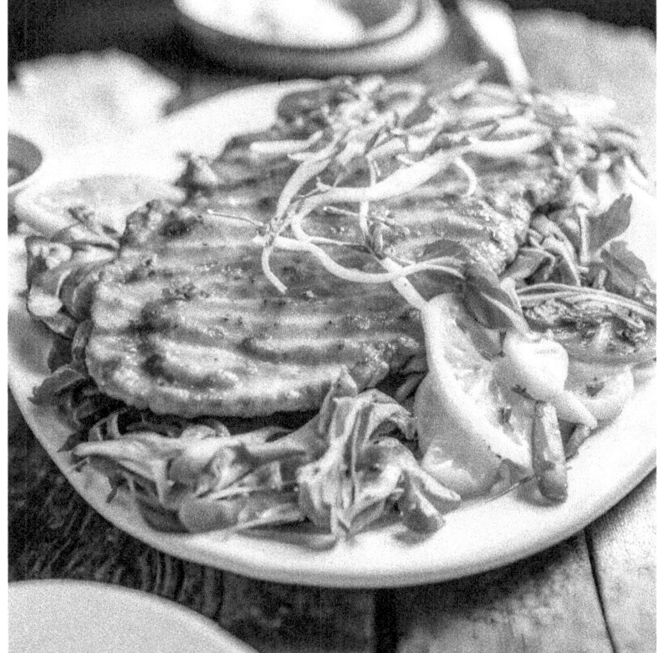

22. Pork Schnitzel

Ingredients

- 4 boneless pork chops
- 1/2 cup gluten-free breadcrumbs
- 1/4 cup gluten-free flour
- 2 large eggs, beaten
- 2 tablespoons olive oil
- 1 tablespoon lemon juice
- 1 tablespoon fresh parsley, chopped (for garnish)

Instructions

1. Place each pork chop between two sheets of plastic wrap and pound with a meat mallet until about 1/4-inch thick.
2. Set up a breading station with three shallow dishes: one with gluten-free flour, one with beaten eggs, and one with gluten-free breadcrumbs.
3. Dredge each pork chop in the flour, dip in the eggs, and coat with breadcrumbs.
4. In a large skillet, heat olive oil over medium-high heat.
5. Add the breaded pork chops and cook for 3-4 minutes on each side until golden brown and cooked through.
6. Remove from heat and drizzle with lemon juice. Garnish with fresh parsley before serving.

Nutrition Info per Serving

- Calories: 350
- Protein: 30g
- Carbohydrates: 20g
- Fat: 15g
- Fiber: 2g

Serves

- 4

Cooking Time

- 20 minutes

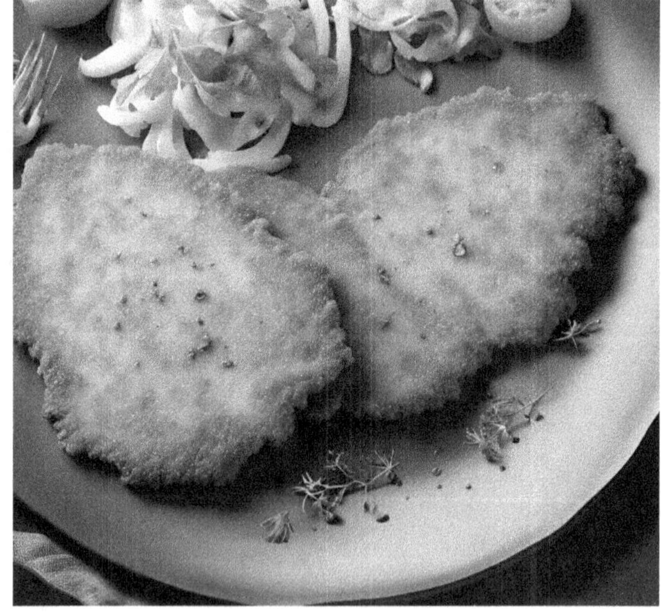

23. Pork Piccata

Ingredients

- 4 boneless pork chops
- 1/4 cup gluten-free flour
- 2 tablespoons olive oil
- 1/2 cup chicken broth
- 1/4 cup lemon juice
- 2 tablespoons capers, drained
- 1 tablespoon fresh parsley, chopped (for garnish)

Instructions

1. Place each pork chop between two sheets of plastic wrap and pound with a meat mallet until about 1/4-inch thick.
2. Dredge the pork chops in gluten-free flour.
3. In a large skillet, heat olive oil over medium-high heat.
4. Add the pork chops and cook for 3-4 minutes on each side until golden brown and cooked through. Remove from skillet and set aside.
5. In the same skillet, add chicken broth, lemon juice, and capers. Bring to a boil, scraping up any browned bits from the bottom of the skillet.
6. Return the pork chops to the skillet and simmer for 2-3 minutes until heated through.
7. Garnish with fresh parsley before serving.

Nutrition Info per Serving

- Calories: 280
- Protein: 28g
- Carbohydrates: 10g
- Fat: 14g
- Fiber: 1g

Serves

- 4

Cooking Time

- 20 minutes

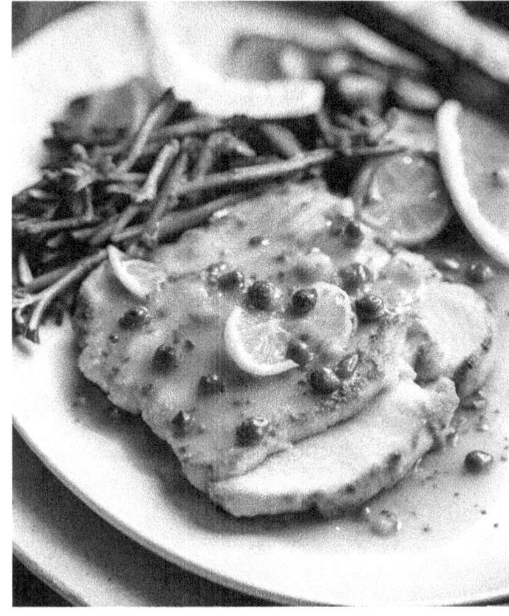

24. Beef Yakitori

Ingredients

- 1 pound beef sirloin, cut into bite-sized pieces
- 1/4 cup low-sodium tamari (gluten-free soy sauce)
- 1/4 cup mirin (sweet rice wine)
- 1 tablespoon sake
- 1 tablespoon brown sugar
- 1 teaspoon garlic-infused oil
- 1 teaspoon grated ginger
- 8 bamboo skewers (soaked in water for 30 minutes)
- 2 green onions, cut into 1-inch pieces

Instructions

1. In a large bowl, combine tamari, mirin, sake, brown sugar, garlic-infused oil, and grated ginger.
2. Add the beef pieces to the marinade and mix until well coated. Marinate in the refrigerator for at least 1 hour.
3. Preheat your grill or grill pan to medium-high heat.
4. Thread the marinated beef pieces and green onion pieces onto the soaked bamboo skewers.
5. Grill the skewers for 2-3 minutes on each side, until the beef is cooked to your desired level of doneness.
6. Serve immediately.

Nutrition Info per Serving

- Calories: 220
- Protein: 25g
- Carbohydrates: 8g
- Fat: 10g
- Fiber: 0g

Serves

- 4

Cooking Time

- 20 minutes (plus marinating time)

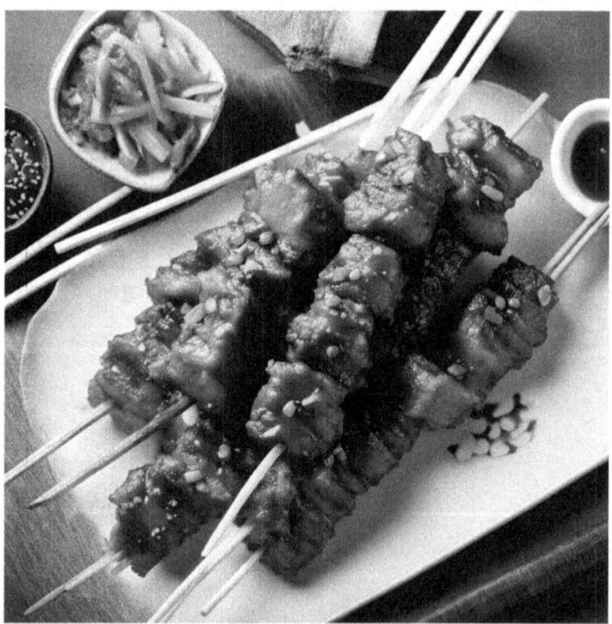

Poultry Recipes

1. Barbecue Chicken Pizza
Ingredients
- 1 gluten-free pizza crust
- 1/2 cup low FODMAP barbecue sauce
- 1 cup cooked chicken breast, shredded
- 1/2 red bell pepper, thinly sliced
- 1/2 cup lactose-free mozzarella cheese, shredded
- 1/4 cup fresh cilantro, chopped

Instructions
1. Preheat your oven according to the pizza crust instructions.
2. Spread the barbecue sauce evenly over the gluten-free pizza crust.
3. Top with shredded chicken, red bell pepper slices, and shredded mozzarella cheese.
4. Bake the pizza in the oven as per the crust instructions (usually about 10-15 minutes) until the cheese is melted and bubbly.
5. Remove from the oven and sprinkle with chopped cilantro before serving.

Nutrition Info per Serving
- Calories: 320
- Protein: 22g
- Carbohydrates: 28g
- Fat: 12g
- Fiber: 3g

Serves
- 4

Cooking Time
- 20 minutes

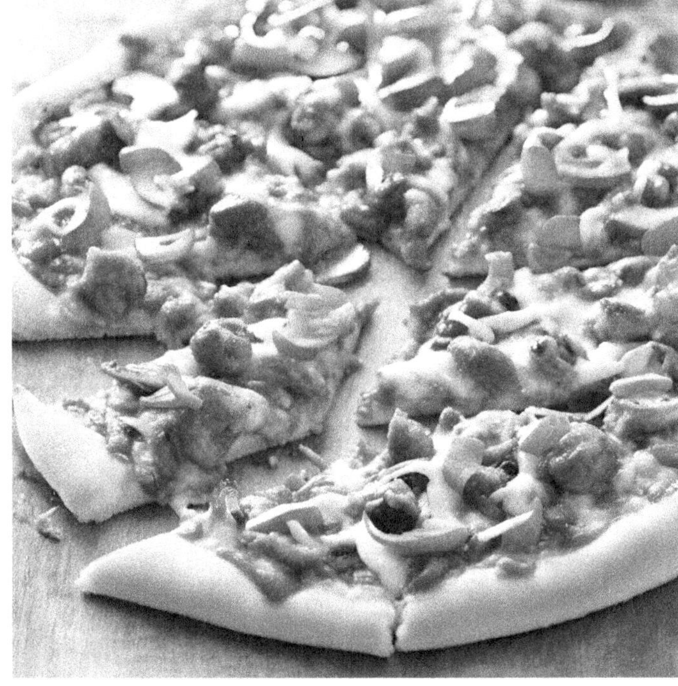

2. Chicken Shawarma

Ingredients

- 1 pound boneless, skinless chicken thighs
- 2 tablespoons olive oil
- 1 tablespoon lemon juice
- 1 teaspoon ground cumin
- 1 teaspoon ground coriander
- 1 teaspoon paprika
- 1/2 teaspoon turmeric
- 1/2 teaspoon ground ginger
- 1/4 teaspoon ground cinnamon
- 1/4 teaspoon ground allspice
- 4 gluten-free pita breads
- 1/2 cup lactose-free yogurt
- 1/2 cucumber, diced
- 1 tablespoon fresh dill, chopped

Instructions

1. In a large bowl, combine olive oil, lemon juice, cumin, coriander, paprika, turmeric, ginger, cinnamon, and allspice. Mix well.
2. Add the chicken thighs to the bowl and coat them evenly with the marinade. Let marinate in the refrigerator for at least 1 hour.
3. Preheat the grill or a grill pan over medium-high heat.
4. Grill the chicken thighs for 5-7 minutes on each side until fully cooked.
5. Let the chicken rest for a few minutes before slicing.
6. In a small bowl, mix the lactose-free yogurt with the diced cucumber and fresh dill.
7. Serve the sliced chicken in gluten-free pita breads, topped with the yogurt sauce.

Nutrition Info per Serving

- Calories: 360
- Protein: 30g
- Carbohydrates: 30g
- Fat: 15g
- Fiber: 4g

Serves

- 4

Cooking Time

- 25 minutes (plus marinating time)

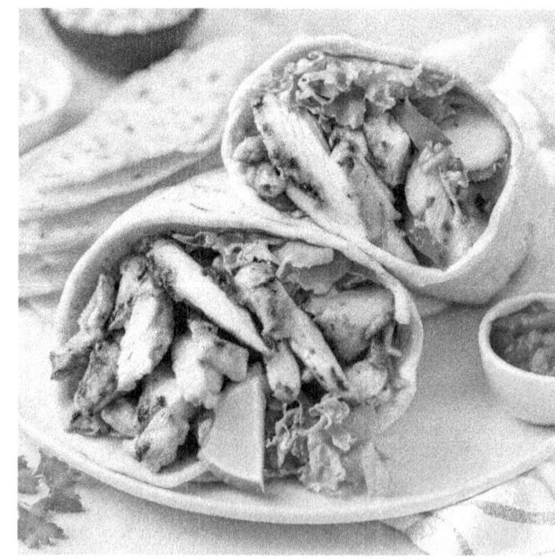

3. Duck Confit

Ingredients

- 4 duck legs
- 1 tablespoon garlic-infused oil
- 1 tablespoon fresh thyme leaves
- 1 teaspoon ground allspice
- 1/4 teaspoon ground cloves
- 1/4 cup duck fat or olive oil

Instructions

1. Preheat your oven to 225°F (110°C).
2. Rub the duck legs with garlic-infused oil, thyme, allspice, and cloves. Let them marinate for at least 1 hour or overnight in the refrigerator.
3. Place the duck legs in an oven-safe dish and pour the duck fat or olive oil over them.
4. Cover the dish with aluminum foil and bake for 2.5 to 3 hours until the meat is tender and falling off the bone.
5. Remove the foil and increase the oven temperature to 400°F (200°C). Bake for an additional 15 minutes until the skin is crispy.
6. Let the duck legs rest for 10 minutes before serving.

Nutrition Info per Serving

- Calories: 450
- Protein: 24g
- Carbohydrates: 1g
- Fat: 38g
- Fiber: 0g

Serves

- 4

Cooking Time

- 3 hours 30 minutes (plus marinating time)

4. Chicken and Vegetable Kebabs

Ingredients

- 1 pound boneless, skinless chicken breast, cut into 1-inch cubes
- 1 red bell pepper, cut into 1-inch pieces
- 1 yellow bell pepper, cut into 1-inch pieces
- 1 zucchini, sliced into rounds
- 1/2 cup cherry tomatoes
- 1/4 cup olive oil
- 2 tablespoons lemon juice
- 1 teaspoon dried oregano
- 1 teaspoon paprika
- 1 teaspoon garlic-infused oil
- Wooden skewers (soaked in water for 30 minutes)

Instructions

1. In a large bowl, combine olive oil, lemon juice, oregano, paprika, and garlic-infused oil.
2. Add the chicken cubes to the bowl and coat them evenly with the marinade. Let marinate in the refrigerator for at least 30 minutes.
3. Preheat the grill or a grill pan over medium-high heat.
4. Thread the marinated chicken, bell peppers, zucchini, and cherry tomatoes onto the soaked wooden skewers.
5. Grill the kebabs for 4-5 minutes on each side until the chicken is cooked through and the vegetables are tender.
6. Serve immediately.

Nutrition Info per Serving

- Calories: 250
- Protein: 28g
- Carbohydrates: 10g
- Fat: 12g
- Fiber: 3g

Serves

- 4

Cooking Time

- 20 minutes (plus marinating time)

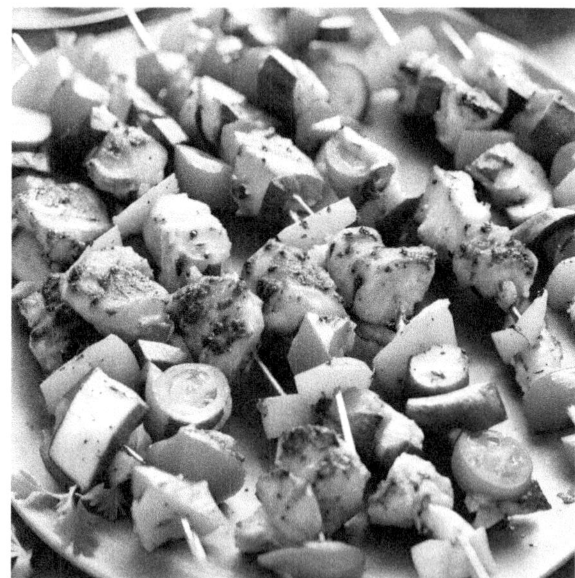

5. Lemon Garlic Turkey Cutlets

Ingredients

- 1 pound turkey cutlets
- 2 tablespoons olive oil
- 2 tablespoons lemon juice
- 1 tablespoon garlic-infused oil
- 1 teaspoon dried oregano
- 1 teaspoon dried thyme
- 1 lemon, sliced

Instructions

1. In a small bowl, mix together olive oil, lemon juice, garlic-infused oil, oregano, and thyme.
2. Coat the turkey cutlets with the marinade and let them sit for at least 15 minutes.
3. Preheat a non-stick skillet over medium-high heat.
4. Add the turkey cutlets and cook for 3-4 minutes on each side until fully cooked and golden brown.
5. Serve the turkey cutlets with lemon slices.

Nutrition Info per Serving

- Calories: 220
- Protein: 30g
- Carbohydrates: 2g
- Fat: 10g
- Fiber: 1g

Serves

- 4

Cooking Time

- 15 minutes (plus marinating time)

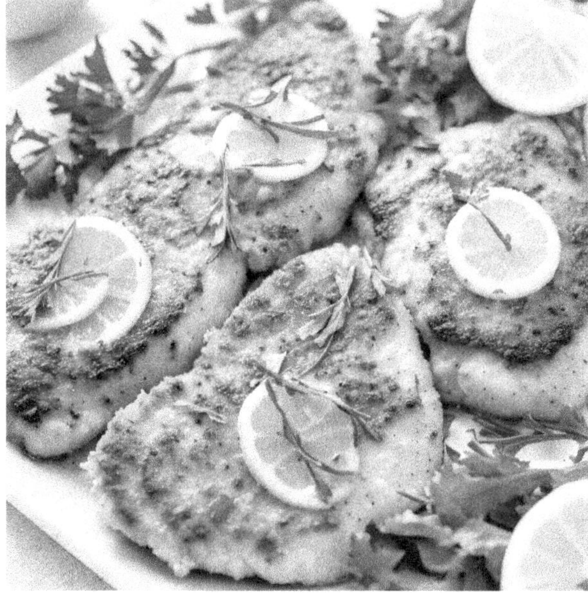

6. Chicken and Broccoli Stir-fry

Ingredients

- 1 pound boneless, skinless chicken breast, sliced thin
- 2 cups broccoli florets
- 1 red bell pepper, sliced
- 2 tablespoons olive oil
- 1 tablespoon garlic-infused oil
- 2 tablespoons low-sodium tamari (gluten-free soy sauce)
- 1 tablespoon oyster sauce (gluten-free)
- 1 teaspoon grated ginger

Instructions

1. Heat olive oil in a large skillet or wok over medium-high heat.
2. Add the chicken slices and cook until browned and cooked through, about 5-7 minutes.
3. Remove the chicken from the skillet and set aside.
4. In the same skillet, add garlic-infused oil, broccoli florets, and red bell pepper. Stir-fry for 3-4 minutes until the vegetables are tender-crisp.
5. Return the chicken to the skillet.
6. In a small bowl, mix together tamari, oyster sauce, and grated ginger. Pour over the chicken and vegetables, and stir to combine.
7. Cook for another 2-3 minutes until everything is heated through.
8. Serve immediately.

Nutrition Info per Serving

- Calories: 250
- Protein: 30g
- Carbohydrates: 10g
- Fat: 10g
- Fiber: 3g

Serves

- 4

Cooking Time

- 20 minutes

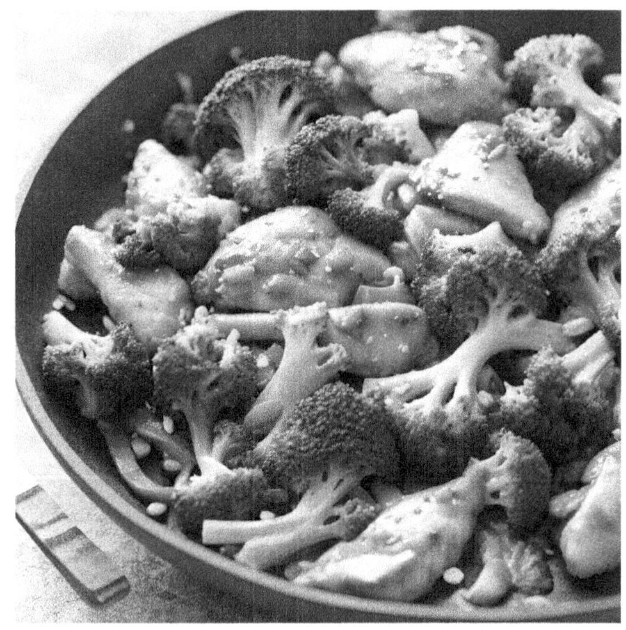

7. Turkey Stuffed Bell Peppers

Ingredients

- 4 bell peppers (any color)
- 1 pound ground turkey
- 1 tablespoon olive oil
- 1 onion, diced
- 1 cup cooked quinoa
- 1 cup diced tomatoes (canned, no added salt)
- 1 teaspoon dried oregano
- 1 teaspoon dried basil
- 1/2 cup lactose-free cheese, shredded (optional)

Instructions

1. Preheat your oven to 375°F (190°C).
2. Cut the tops off the bell peppers and remove the seeds and membranes.
3. In a large skillet, heat olive oil over medium heat.
4. Add the diced onion and cook until softened, about 5 minutes.
5. Add the ground turkey and cook until browned, about 7-8 minutes.
6. Stir in the cooked quinoa, diced tomatoes, oregano, and basil. Cook for another 2-3 minutes until heated through.
7. Stuff the bell peppers with the turkey mixture and place them in a baking dish.
8. If using, sprinkle shredded cheese on top of the stuffed peppers.
9. Cover with aluminum foil and bake for 30 minutes. Remove the foil and bake for an additional 10 minutes until the peppers are tender.
10. Serve immediately.

Nutrition Info per Serving

- Calories: 300
- Protein: 25g
- Carbohydrates: 20g
- Fat: 12g
- Fiber: 5g

Serves

- 4

Cooking Time

- 45 minutes

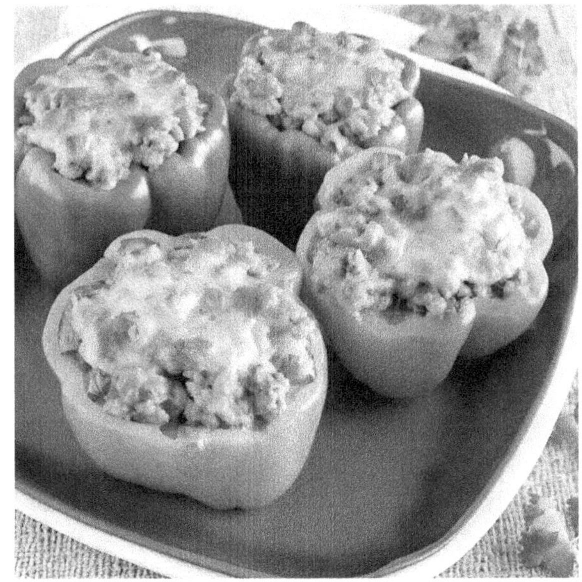

8. Chicken Cacciatore

Ingredients

- 1 pound boneless, skinless chicken thighs
- 2 tablespoons olive oil
- 1 onion, diced
- 2 garlic-infused oil
- 1 red bell pepper, sliced
- 1 cup diced tomatoes (canned, no added salt)
- 1/2 cup chicken broth
- 1 teaspoon dried oregano
- 1 teaspoon dried basil
- 1/4 cup fresh parsley, chopped

Instructions

1. In a large skillet, heat olive oil over medium-high heat.
2. Add the chicken thighs and cook until browned on both sides, about 5-7 minutes per side. Remove the chicken and set aside.
3. In the same skillet, add the diced onion and cook until softened, about 5 minutes.
4. Add garlic-infused oil and red bell pepper. Cook for another 3-4 minutes.
5. Stir in the diced tomatoes, chicken broth, oregano, and basil. Bring to a simmer.
6. Return the chicken to the skillet and cover. Simmer for 20-25 minutes until the chicken is cooked through and tender.
7. Garnish with fresh parsley before serving.

Nutrition Info per Serving

- Calories: 280
- Protein: 25g
- Carbohydrates: 12g
- Fat: 14g
- Fiber: 3g

Serves

- 4

Cooking Time

- 40 minutes

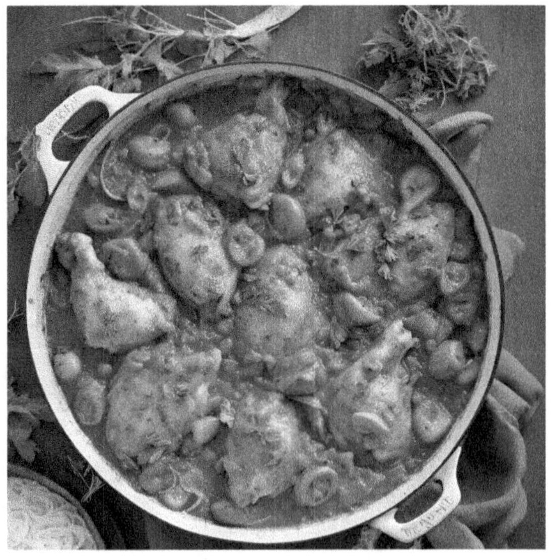

9. Turkey Soup

Ingredients

- 1 pound cooked turkey breast, shredded
- 1 onion, diced
- 2 carrots, sliced
- 2 celery stalks, sliced
- 1 zucchini, diced
- 8 cups chicken or turkey broth (low sodium)
- 2 tablespoons olive oil
- 1 teaspoon dried thyme
- 1 teaspoon dried rosemary
- 1/2 cup cooked quinoa (optional)

Instructions

1. In a large pot, heat olive oil over medium heat.
2. Add the diced onion, carrots, and celery. Cook until the vegetables are softened, about 5 minutes.
3. Add the diced zucchini and cook for another 3-4 minutes.
4. Pour in the broth and bring to a boil.
5. Add the shredded turkey, thyme, and rosemary. Reduce heat and simmer for 20 minutes.
6. Stir in the cooked quinoa if using, and cook for another 5 minutes until heated through.
7. Serve hot.

Nutrition Info per Serving

- Calories: 200
- Protein: 20g
- Carbohydrates: 12g
- Fat: 8g
- Fiber: 3g

Serves

- 6

Cooking Time

- 35 minutes

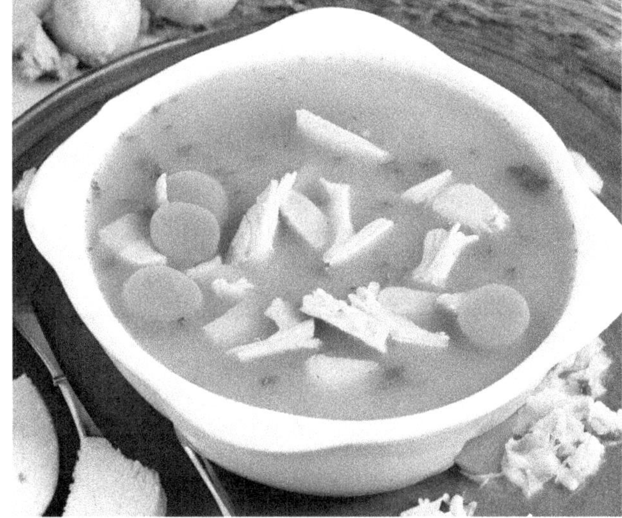

10. Chicken Piccata

Ingredients

- 4 boneless, skinless chicken breasts
- 1/4 cup gluten-free flour
- 2 tablespoons olive oil
- 1/4 cup chicken broth (low sodium)
- 1/4 cup lemon juice
- 2 tablespoons capers, drained
- 1 tablespoon garlic-infused oil
- 1 tablespoon fresh parsley, chopped (for garnish)

Instructions

1. Pound the chicken breasts to 1/4-inch thickness and dredge them in gluten-free flour.
2. In a large skillet, heat olive oil over medium-high heat.
3. Add the chicken breasts and cook for 3-4 minutes on each side until golden brown and cooked through. Remove from skillet and set aside.
4. In the same skillet, add chicken broth, lemon juice, capers, and garlic-infused oil. Bring to a boil, scraping up any browned bits from the bottom of the skillet.
5. Return the chicken breasts to the skillet and simmer for 2-3 minutes until heated through.
6. Garnish with fresh parsley before serving.

Nutrition Info per Serving

- Calories: 280
- Protein: 30g
- Carbohydrates: 10g
- Fat: 12g
- Fiber: 1g

Serves

- 4

Cooking Time

- 20 minutes

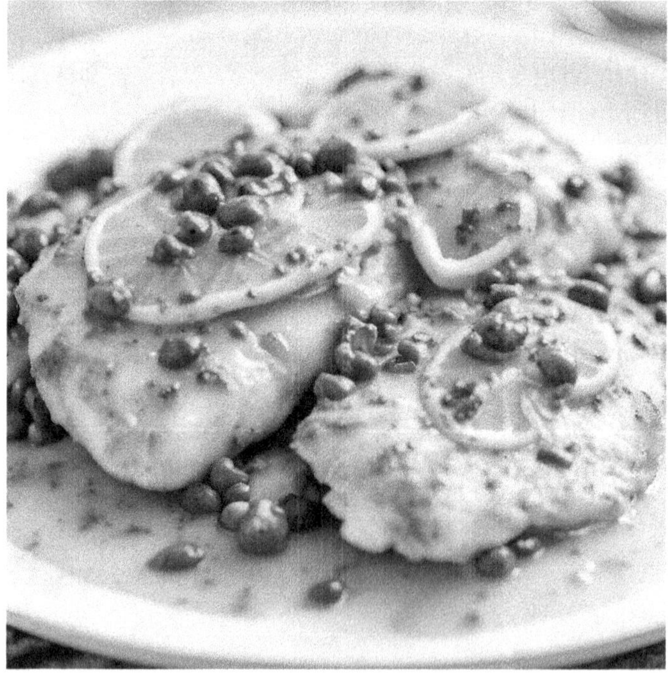

11. Chicken Parmesan

Ingredients

- 4 boneless, skinless chicken breasts
- 1/2 cup gluten-free breadcrumbs
- 1/4 cup gluten-free flour
- 2 large eggs, beaten
- 2 tablespoons olive oil
- 1 cup marinara sauce (low FODMAP)
- 1 cup lactose-free mozzarella cheese, shredded
- 1/4 cup grated Parmesan cheese
- 1 tablespoon fresh basil, chopped (for garnish)

Instructions

1. Preheat your oven to 375°F (190°C).
2. Pound the chicken breasts to 1/2-inch thickness. Set up a breading station with three shallow dishes: one with gluten-free flour, one with beaten eggs, and one with gluten-free breadcrumbs.
3. Dredge each chicken breast in the flour, dip in the eggs, and coat with breadcrumbs.
4. In a large skillet, heat olive oil over medium-high heat. Add the breaded chicken breasts and cook for 3-4 minutes on each side until golden brown.
5. Place the chicken breasts in a baking dish. Top each with marinara sauce, mozzarella cheese, and Parmesan cheese.
6. Bake for 20 minutes until the cheese is melted and bubbly.
7. Garnish with fresh basil before serving.

Nutrition Info per Serving

- Calories: 400
- Protein: 36g
- Carbohydrates: 20g
- Fat: 18g
- Fiber: 2g

Serves

- 4

Cooking Time

- 35 minutes

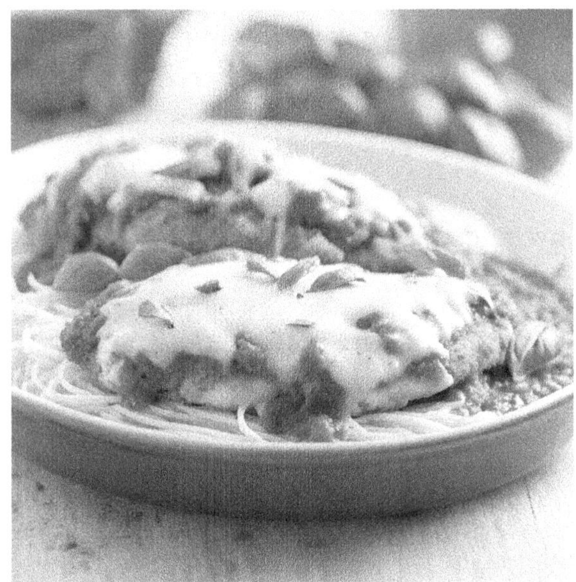

12. Chicken Paella

Ingredients

- 1 pound boneless, skinless chicken thighs, cut into bite-sized pieces
- 2 tablespoons olive oil
- 1 red bell pepper, diced
- 1 green bell pepper, diced
- 1 cup long-grain rice
- 2 cups chicken broth (low sodium)
- 1/2 cup diced tomatoes (canned, no added salt)
- 1 teaspoon smoked paprika
- 1/2 teaspoon turmeric
- 1/2 cup frozen peas
- 1/4 cup fresh parsley, chopped (for garnish)
- 1 lemon, cut into wedges (for serving)

Instructions

1. In a large skillet or paella pan, heat olive oil over medium-high heat.
2. Add the chicken pieces and cook until browned, about 5-7 minutes. Remove and set aside.
3. In the same pan, add the diced red and green bell peppers. Cook until softened, about 5 minutes.
4. Stir in the rice, smoked paprika, and turmeric. Cook for 1-2 minutes to toast the rice.
5. Add the chicken broth and diced tomatoes. Bring to a boil, then reduce heat to low and simmer for 15 minutes.
6. Return the chicken to the pan and stir in the frozen peas. Cook for another 5-7 minutes until the rice is tender and the liquid is absorbed.
7. Garnish with fresh parsley and serve with lemon wedges.

Nutrition Info per Serving

- Calories: 350
- Protein: 28g
- Carbohydrates: 40g
- Fat: 10g
- Fiber: 4g

Serves

- 4

Cooking Time

- 40 minutes

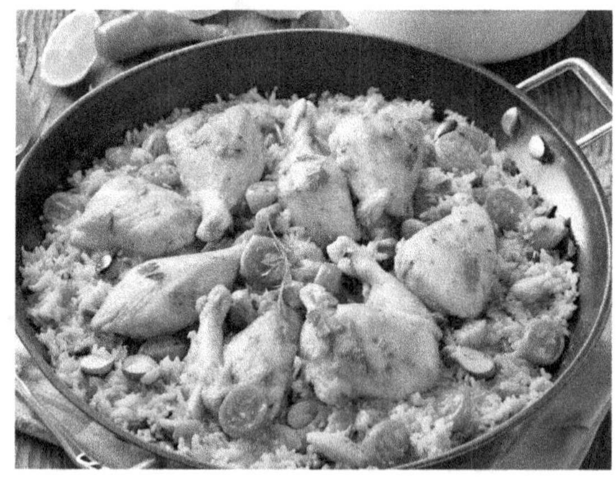

13. Turkey and Spinach Meatloaf

Ingredients

- 1 pound ground turkey
- 1 cup fresh spinach, chopped
- 1/2 cup gluten-free breadcrumbs
- 1/4 cup lactose-free milk
- 1 egg
- 1 onion, finely diced
- 1 tablespoon Worcestershire sauce (gluten-free)
- 1 teaspoon dried thyme

Instructions

1. Preheat your oven to 375°F (190°C).
2. In a large bowl, combine ground turkey, chopped spinach, gluten-free breadcrumbs, lactose-free milk, egg, diced onion, Worcestershire sauce, and thyme. Mix until well combined.
3. Transfer the mixture to a loaf pan and shape it into a loaf.
4. Bake for 45 minutes until the meatloaf is cooked through and the internal temperature reaches 165°F (74°C).
5. Let the meatloaf rest for 10 minutes before slicing and serving.

Nutrition Info per Serving

- Calories: 250
- Protein: 24g
- Carbohydrates: 15g
- Fat: 12g
- Fiber: 2g

Serves

- 4

Cooking Time

- 55 minutes

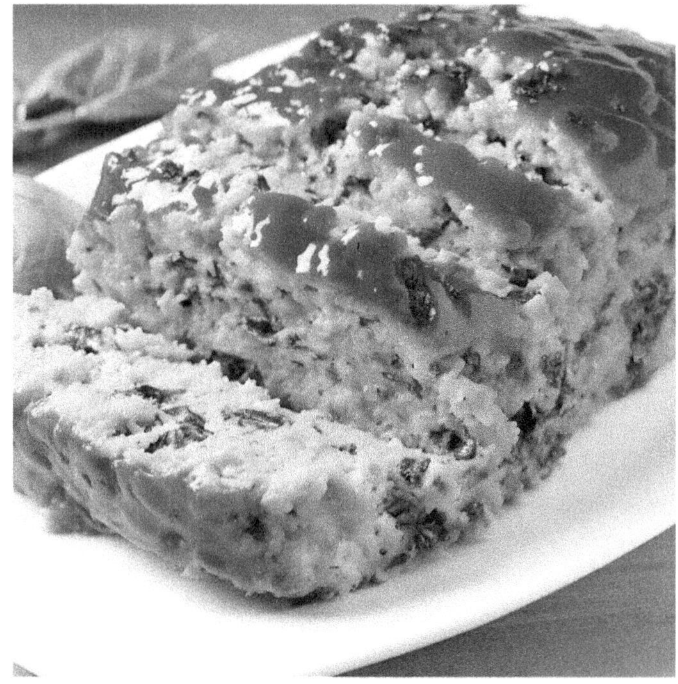

14. Roasted Chicken Thighs

Ingredients

- 1 pound bone-in, skin-on chicken thighs
- 2 tablespoons olive oil
- 1 tablespoon garlic-infused oil
- 1 tablespoon lemon juice
- 1 teaspoon dried rosemary
- 1 teaspoon dried thyme

Instructions

1. Preheat your oven to 400°F (200°C).
2. In a small bowl, mix together olive oil, garlic-infused oil, lemon juice, rosemary, and thyme.
3. Rub the mixture all over the chicken thighs.
4. Place the chicken thighs on a baking sheet, skin side up.
5. Roast in the preheated oven for 35-40 minutes until the skin is crispy and the chicken is cooked through.
6. Let the chicken rest for 5 minutes before serving.

Nutrition Info per Serving

- Calories: 300
- Protein: 24g
- Carbohydrates: 2g
- Fat: 22g
- Fiber: 1g

Serves

- 4

Cooking Time

- 45 minutes

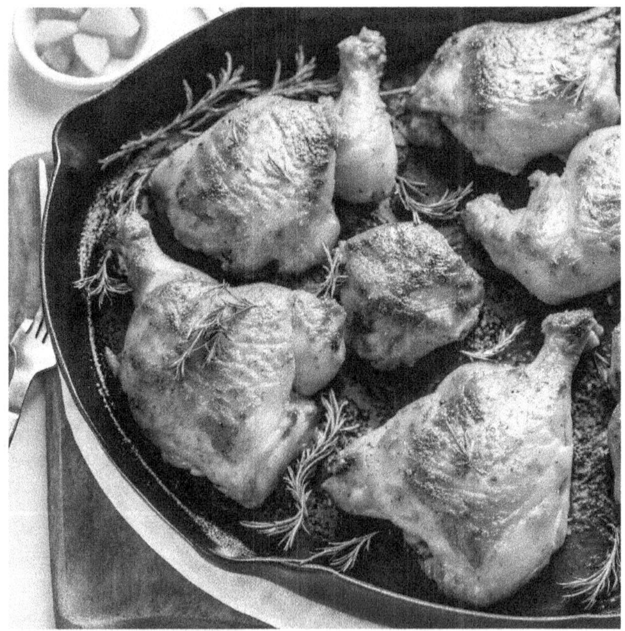

15. Grilled Chicken Skewers

Ingredients

- 1 pound boneless, skinless chicken breast, cut into 1-inch cubes
- 2 tablespoons olive oil
- 1 tablespoon lemon juice
- 1 teaspoon garlic-infused oil
- 1 teaspoon dried oregano
- 1/2 teaspoon smoked paprika
- 1 red bell pepper, cut into 1-inch pieces
- 1 yellow bell pepper, cut into 1-inch pieces
- 1 zucchini, sliced into rounds
- Wooden skewers (soaked in water for 30 minutes)

Instructions

1. In a large bowl, combine olive oil, lemon juice, garlic-infused oil, oregano, and smoked paprika.
2. Add the chicken cubes to the bowl and coat them evenly with the marinade. Let marinate in the refrigerator for at least 30 minutes.
3. Preheat the grill or grill pan to medium-high heat.
4. Thread the marinated chicken, red bell pepper, yellow bell pepper, and zucchini onto the soaked wooden skewers.
5. Grill the skewers for 4-5 minutes on each side until the chicken is cooked through and the vegetables are tender.
6. Serve immediately.

Nutrition Info per Serving

- Calories: 250
- Protein: 28g
- Carbohydrates: 8g
- Fat: 12g
- Fiber: 3g

Serves

- 4

Cooking Time

- 20 minutes (plus marinating time)

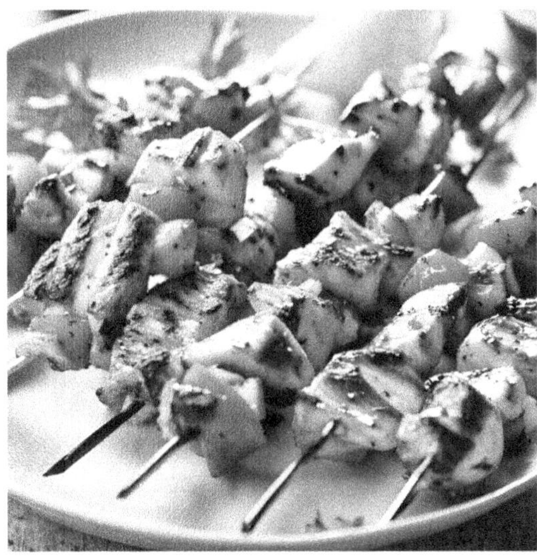

16. Pulled Turkey Sandwich

Ingredients

- 1 pound cooked turkey breast, shredded
- 1/2 cup low FODMAP barbecue sauce
- 4 gluten-free buns
- 1/2 cup coleslaw (optional, low FODMAP)

Instructions

1. In a large bowl, combine shredded turkey and barbecue sauce. Mix until well coated.
2. Heat the turkey mixture in a skillet over medium heat until warmed through, about 5 minutes.
3. Serve the pulled turkey on gluten-free buns with a side of coleslaw, if desired.

Nutrition Info per Serving

- Calories: 300
- Protein: 28g
- Carbohydrates: 30g
- Fat: 8g
- Fiber: 3g

Serves

- 4

Cooking Time

- 10 minutes

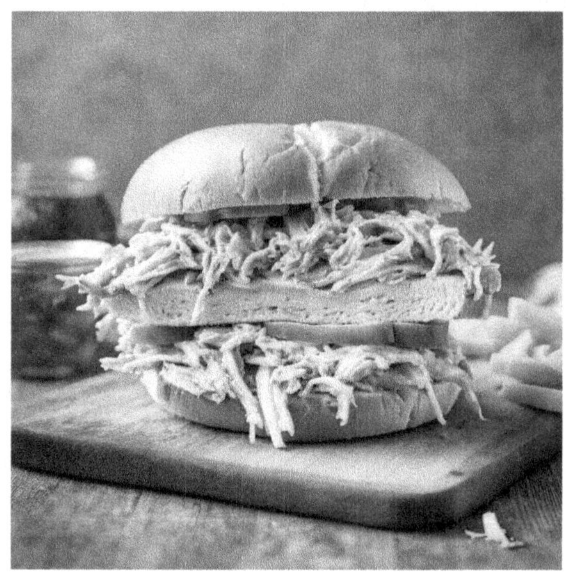

17. Chicken Curry

Ingredients

- 1 pound boneless, skinless chicken breast, cut into bite-sized pieces
- 2 tablespoons olive oil
- 1 onion, diced
- 1 tablespoon garlic-infused oil
- 1 tablespoon grated ginger
- 1 tablespoon curry powder
- 1 cup coconut milk (canned)
- 1 cup chicken broth (low sodium)
- 1 cup diced tomatoes (canned, no added salt)
- 2 cups spinach, chopped

Instructions

1. In a large pot, heat olive oil over medium-high heat.
2. Add the diced onion and cook until softened, about 5 minutes.
3. Add garlic-infused oil, grated ginger, and curry powder. Cook for another 1-2 minutes until fragrant.
4. Add the chicken pieces and cook until browned, about 5-7 minutes.
5. Stir in the coconut milk, chicken broth, and diced tomatoes. Bring to a simmer.
6. Reduce heat and cook for 20 minutes until the chicken is cooked through and the sauce has thickened.
7. Stir in the chopped spinach and cook for another 2-3 minutes until wilted.
8. Serve hot.

Nutrition Info per Serving

- Calories: 350
- Protein: 30g
- Carbohydrates: 12g
- Fat: 20g
- Fiber: 4g

Serves

- 4

Cooking Time

- 35 minutes

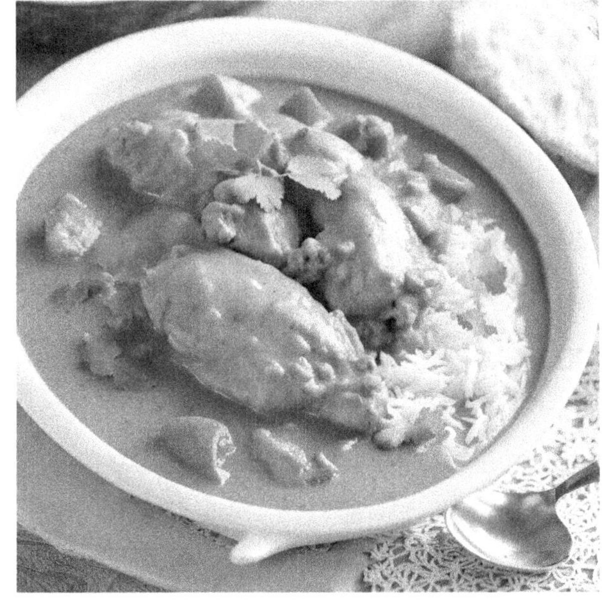

18. Chicken Risotto

Ingredients

- 1 pound boneless, skinless chicken breast, cut into bite-sized pieces
- 2 tablespoons olive oil
- 1 onion, diced
- 1 cup Arborio rice
- 1/2 cup dry white wine (optional)
- 4 cups chicken broth (low sodium), warmed
- 1 cup peas (frozen or fresh)
- 1/2 cup Parmesan cheese, grated
- 1 tablespoon garlic-infused oil
- 1 tablespoon fresh parsley, chopped (for garnish)

Instructions

1. In a large pot or Dutch oven, heat olive oil over medium-high heat.
2. Add the chicken pieces and cook until browned, about 5-7 minutes. Remove from the pot and set aside.
3. In the same pot, add the diced onion and cook until softened, about 5 minutes.
4. Stir in the Arborio rice and cook for 1-2 minutes until lightly toasted.
5. Pour in the white wine (if using) and cook until mostly absorbed.
6. Add the warm chicken broth, one ladleful at a time, stirring frequently and allowing the liquid to be absorbed before adding more.
7. Continue until the rice is creamy and cooked through, about 20 minutes.
8. Stir in the cooked chicken, peas, Parmesan cheese, and garlic-infused oil.
9. Cook for another 2-3 minutes until everything is heated through.
10. Garnish with fresh parsley before serving.

Nutrition Info per Serving

- Calories: 400
- Protein: 30g
- Carbohydrates: 40g
- Fat: 14g
- Fiber: 3g

Serves

- 4

Cooking Time

- 40 minutes

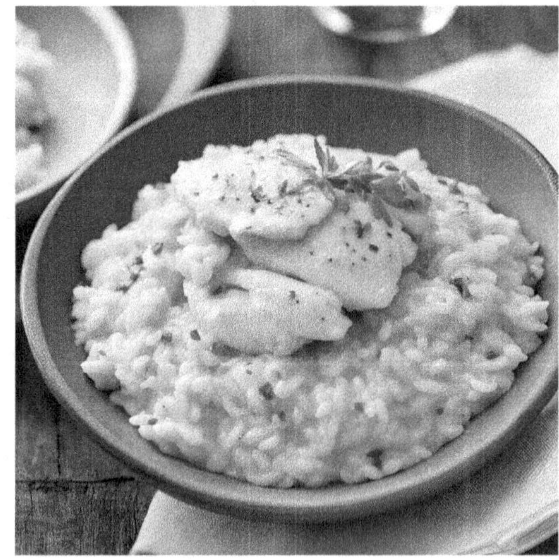

19. Smoked Turkey Breast

Ingredients

- 1 whole turkey breast (about 3 pounds)
- 2 tablespoons olive oil
- 1 tablespoon garlic-infused oil
- 1 tablespoon smoked paprika
- 1 teaspoon dried thyme
- 1 teaspoon dried rosemary
- 1/4 cup apple cider vinegar
- 1/4 cup apple juice

Instructions

1. Preheat your smoker to 225°F (110°C).
2. In a small bowl, mix together olive oil, garlic-infused oil, smoked paprika, thyme, and rosemary.
3. Rub the mixture all over the turkey breast.
4. Place the turkey breast in the smoker and smoke for about 3-4 hours, until the internal temperature reaches 165°F (74°C).
5. In a small bowl, mix together apple cider vinegar and apple juice. Baste the turkey breast with this mixture every hour.
6. Let the turkey breast rest for 10-15 minutes before slicing and serving.

Nutrition Info per Serving

- Calories: 220
- Protein: 35g
- Carbohydrates: 2g
- Fat: 8g
- Fiber: 1g

Serves

- 6

Cooking Time

- 4 hours

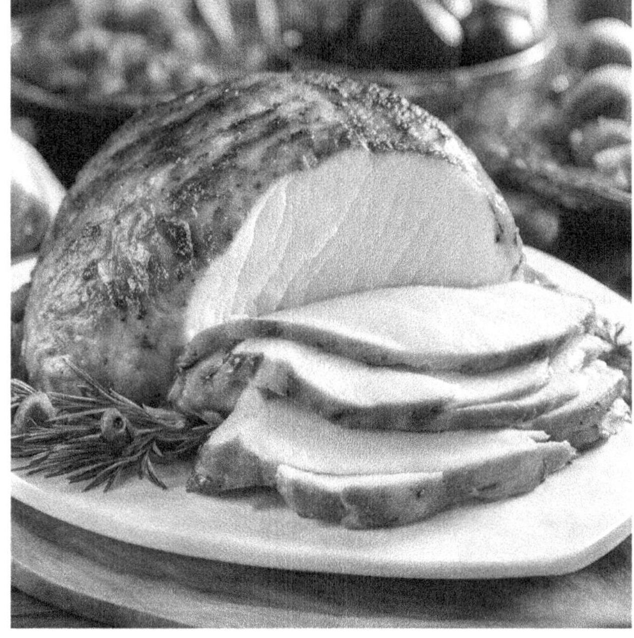

20. Stuffed Chicken Breast

Ingredients

- 4 boneless, skinless chicken breasts
- 1 cup fresh spinach, chopped
- 1/2 cup lactose-free ricotta cheese
- 1/4 cup sun-dried tomatoes, chopped
- 1 tablespoon garlic-infused oil
- 1 teaspoon dried oregano
- 2 tablespoons olive oil

Instructions

1. Preheat your oven to 375°F (190°C).
2. In a bowl, mix together chopped spinach, lactose-free ricotta cheese, sun-dried tomatoes, garlic-infused oil, and dried oregano.
3. Cut a slit in each chicken breast to create a pocket.
4. Stuff each chicken breast with the spinach mixture.
5. Heat olive oil in a large oven-safe skillet over medium-high heat.
6. Sear the stuffed chicken breasts for 3-4 minutes on each side until golden brown.
7. Transfer the skillet to the preheated oven and bake for 20-25 minutes until the chicken is cooked through.
8. Let the chicken rest for 5 minutes before serving.

Nutrition Info per Serving

- Calories: 320
- Protein: 35g
- Carbohydrates: 4g
- Fat: 18g
- Fiber: 2g

Serves

- 4

Cooking Time

- 30 minutes

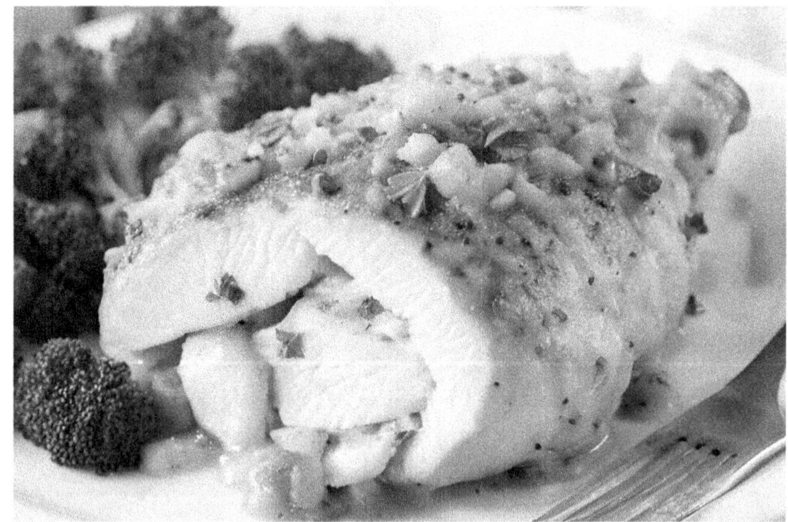

21. Baked Turkey Wings

Ingredients

- 2 pounds turkey wings
- 2 tablespoons olive oil
- 1 tablespoon garlic-infused oil
- 1 teaspoon dried thyme
- 1 teaspoon smoked paprika
- 1/4 cup chicken broth (low sodium)

Instructions

1. Preheat your oven to 375°F (190°C).
2. In a small bowl, mix together olive oil, garlic-infused oil, thyme, and smoked paprika.
3. Rub the mixture all over the turkey wings.
4. Place the turkey wings in a baking dish and pour the chicken broth into the bottom of the dish.
5. Cover the dish with aluminum foil and bake for 45 minutes.
6. Remove the foil and bake for an additional 15 minutes until the skin is crispy.
7. Let the wings rest for 5 minutes before serving.

Nutrition Info per Serving

- Calories: 320
- Protein: 35g
- Carbohydrates: 2g
- Fat: 18g
- Fiber: 1g

Serves

- 4

Cooking Time

- 1 hour

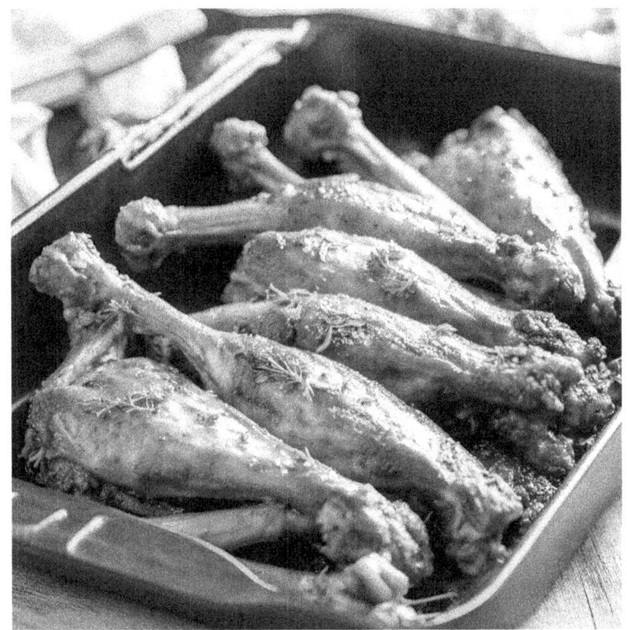

22. Maple Mustard Chicken

Ingredients

- 4 boneless, skinless chicken breasts
- 1/4 cup maple syrup
- 2 tablespoons Dijon mustard
- 1 tablespoon olive oil
- 1 teaspoon garlic-infused oil
- 1 teaspoon dried rosemary

Instructions

1. Preheat your oven to 400°F (200°C).
2. In a small bowl, mix together maple syrup, Dijon mustard, olive oil, garlic-infused oil, and rosemary.
3. Place the chicken breasts in a baking dish and pour the maple mustard mixture over them, turning to coat.
4. Bake for 25-30 minutes until the chicken is cooked through and the glaze is caramelized.
5. Let the chicken rest for 5 minutes before serving.

Nutrition Info per Serving

- Calories: 280
- Protein: 30g
- Carbohydrates: 10g
- Fat: 12g
- Fiber: 1g

Serves

- 4

Cooking Time

- 30 minutes

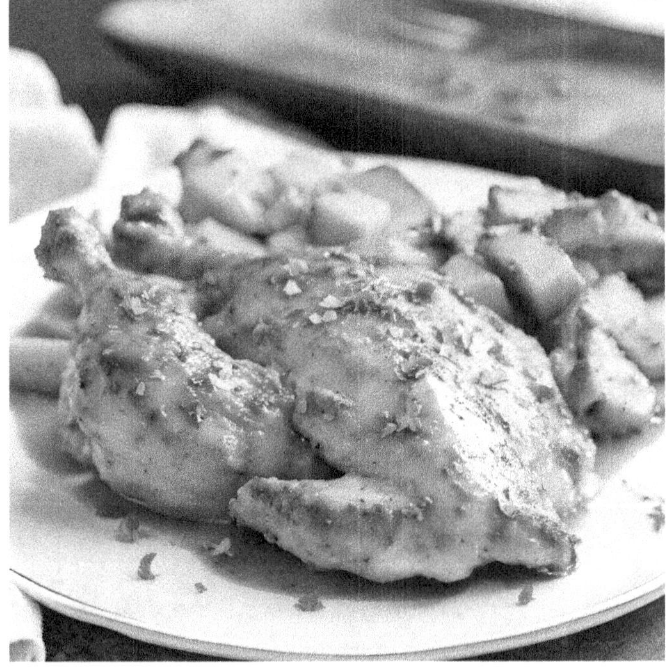

23. Chicken Stir-Fry

Ingredients

- 1 pound boneless, skinless chicken breast, sliced thin
- 2 tablespoons olive oil
- 1 red bell pepper, sliced
- 1 green bell pepper, sliced
- 1 cup broccoli florets
- 1 tablespoon garlic-infused oil
- 2 tablespoons low-sodium tamari (gluten-free soy sauce)
- 1 tablespoon oyster sauce (gluten-free)
- 1 teaspoon grated ginger

Instructions

1. Heat olive oil in a large skillet or wok over medium-high heat.
2. Add the chicken slices and cook until browned and cooked through, about 5-7 minutes.
3. Remove the chicken from the skillet and set aside.
4. In the same skillet, add garlic-infused oil, red bell pepper, green bell pepper, and broccoli. Stir-fry for 3-4 minutes until the vegetables are tender-crisp.
5. Return the chicken to the skillet.
6. In a small bowl, mix together tamari, oyster sauce, and grated ginger. Pour over the chicken and vegetables, and stir to combine.
7. Cook for another 2-3 minutes until everything is heated through.
8. Serve immediately.

Nutrition Info per Serving

- Calories: 260
- Protein: 28g
- Carbohydrates: 10g
- Fat: 12g
- Fiber: 3g

Serves

- 4

Cooking Time

- 20 minutes

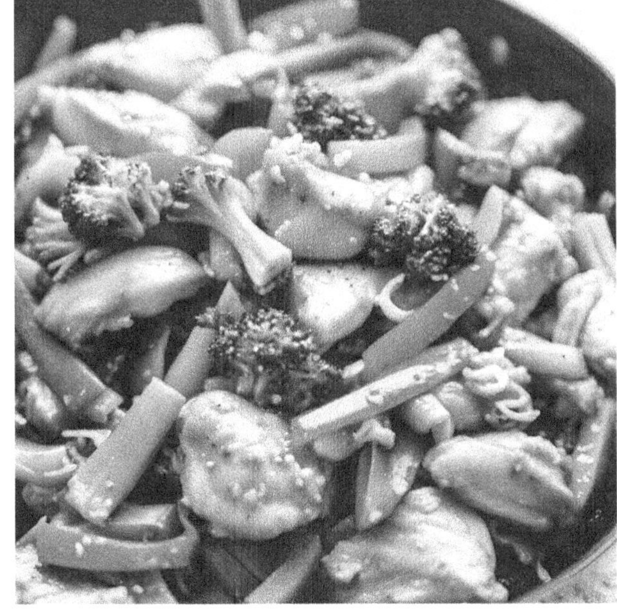

24. Roast Turkey

Ingredients

- 1 whole turkey (10-12 pounds)
- 1/4 cup olive oil
- 2 tablespoons garlic-infused oil
- 2 tablespoons fresh rosemary, chopped
- 2 tablespoons fresh thyme, chopped
- 1/4 cup chicken broth (low sodium)
- 1 lemon, cut into wedges

Instructions

1. Preheat your oven to 325°F (165°C).
2. In a small bowl, mix together olive oil, garlic-infused oil, rosemary, and thyme.
3. Rub the mixture all over the turkey, including under the skin.
4. Place the turkey on a rack in a roasting pan. Pour the chicken broth into the bottom of the pan.
5. Roast the turkey for 3-3.5 hours, or until the internal temperature reaches 165°F (74°C), basting occasionally with the pan juices.
6. Let the turkey rest for 20-30 minutes before carving.
7. Serve with lemon wedges.

Nutrition Info per Serving

- Calories: 350
- Protein: 45g
- Carbohydrates: 2g
- Fat: 18g
- Fiber: 1g

Serves

- 10-12

Cooking Time

- 3.5 hours

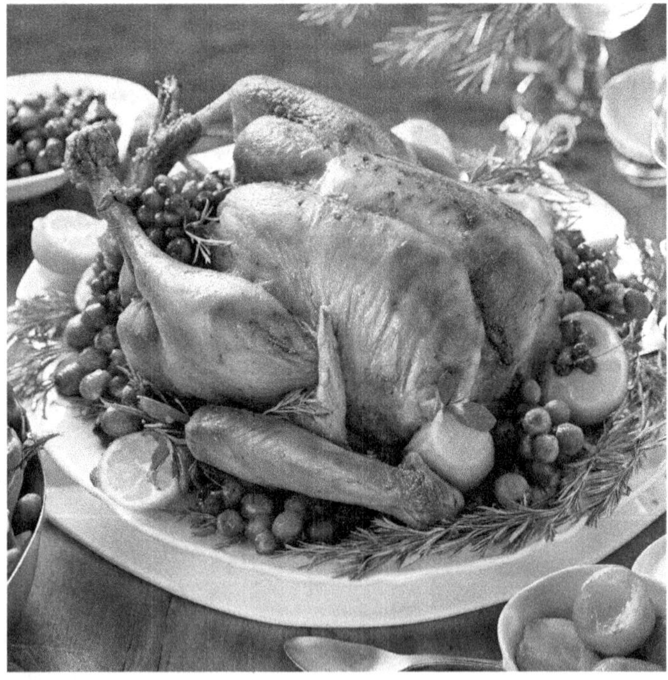

Fish and Seafood

1. Smoked Salmon Breakfast Plate
Ingredients
- 8 ounces smoked salmon
- 4 hard-boiled eggs, sliced
- 1 avocado, sliced
- 1 cup cherry tomatoes, halved
- 1 cucumber, sliced
- 1 tablespoon capers
- 1 tablespoon lemon juice
- 1 tablespoon olive oil
- 1 tablespoon fresh dill, chopped

Instructions
1. Arrange the smoked salmon, hard-boiled eggs, avocado slices, cherry tomatoes, and cucumber slices on a large plate.
2. Sprinkle capers over the top.
3. In a small bowl, mix together lemon juice, olive oil, and chopped dill.
4. Drizzle the dressing over the plate.
5. Serve immediately.

Nutrition Info per Serving
- Calories: 300
- Protein: 20g
- Carbohydrates: 8g
- Fat: 22g
- Fiber: 6g

Serves
- 2

Cooking Time
- 10 minutes

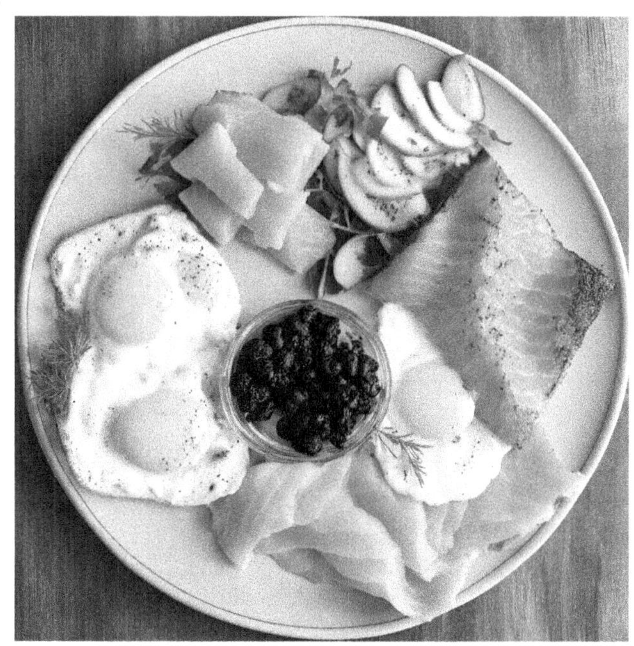

2. Scallops and Asparagus

Ingredients

- 1 pound scallops, patted dry
- 1 bunch asparagus, trimmed
- 2 tablespoons olive oil
- 1 tablespoon garlic-infused oil
- 1 tablespoon lemon juice
- 1 teaspoon dried thyme
- 1 tablespoon fresh parsley, chopped (for garnish)

Instructions

1. Preheat oven to 400°F (200°C).
2. Toss the asparagus with 1 tablespoon of olive oil, garlic-infused oil, and dried thyme. Spread on a baking sheet and roast for 10-12 minutes until tender.
3. While the asparagus is roasting, heat the remaining olive oil in a large skillet over medium-high heat.
4. Add the scallops to the skillet and cook for 2-3 minutes on each side until they are golden brown and cooked through.
5. Remove the asparagus from the oven and transfer to a serving platter.
6. Place the cooked scallops on top of the asparagus.
7. Drizzle with lemon juice and garnish with fresh parsley before serving.

Nutrition Info per Serving

- Calories: 250
- Protein: 25g
- Carbohydrates: 8g
- Fat: 12g
- Fiber: 3g

Serves

- 4

Cooking Time

- 20 minutes

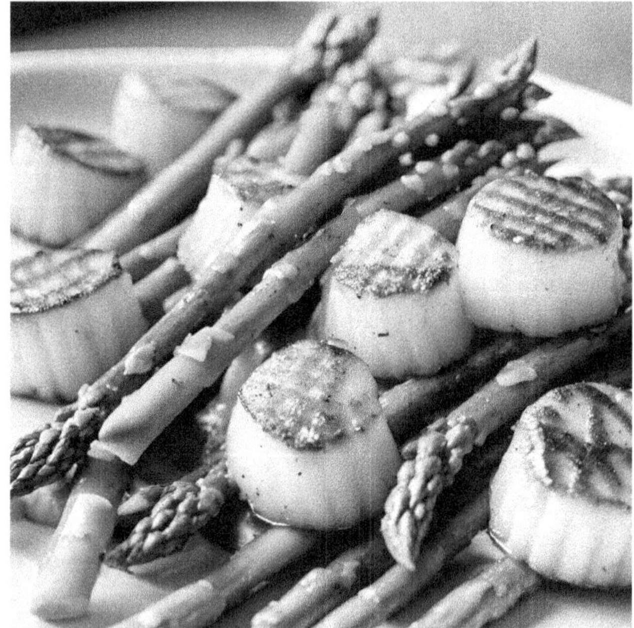

3. Tuna Nicoise Salad

Ingredients

- 2 cans tuna in olive oil, drained
- 4 hard-boiled eggs, quartered
- 1/2 pound green beans, blanched
- 1/2 cup cherry tomatoes, halved
- 1/4 cup black olives
- 1/4 cup capers
- 4 cups mixed salad greens
- 2 tablespoons lemon juice
- 2 tablespoons olive oil
- 1 tablespoon Dijon mustard

Instructions

1. Arrange the salad greens on a large platter.
2. Top with tuna, hard-boiled eggs, green beans, cherry tomatoes, black olives, and capers.
3. In a small bowl, whisk together lemon juice, olive oil, and Dijon mustard.
4. Drizzle the dressing over the salad.
5. Serve immediately.

Nutrition Info per Serving

- Calories: 350
- Protein: 30g
- Carbohydrates: 12g
- Fat: 22g
- Fiber: 5g

Serves

- 4

Cooking Time

- 15 minutes

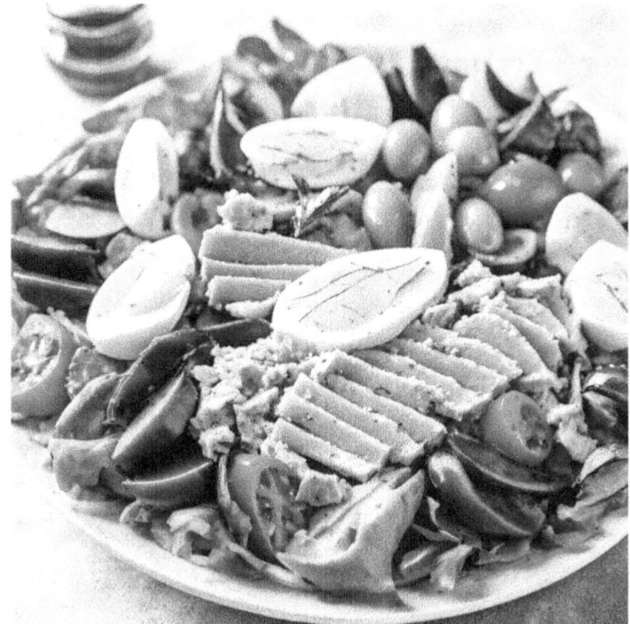

4. Kedgeree

Ingredients

- 1 cup basmati rice
- 1 pound smoked haddock fillets
- 2 cups water
- 4 hard-boiled eggs, chopped
- 1/4 cup lactose-free butter
- 1 tablespoon garlic-infused oil
- 1 tablespoon curry powder
- 1/4 cup fresh parsley, chopped
- 1 tablespoon lemon juice

Instructions

1. Rinse the basmati rice under cold water until the water runs clear.
2. In a large pot, bring 2 cups of water to a boil. Add the rice, reduce heat to low, cover, and cook for 15 minutes until the rice is tender.
3. Meanwhile, in a large skillet, bring about an inch of water to a simmer. Add the smoked haddock fillets and poach for 5-7 minutes until cooked through. Remove the fish, flake it, and set aside.
4. In the same skillet, melt the butter and add the garlic-infused oil and curry powder. Cook for 1 minute until fragrant.
5. Add the cooked rice and flaked haddock to the skillet. Stir to combine and heat through.
6. Gently fold in the chopped hard-boiled eggs and parsley.
7. Drizzle with lemon juice before serving.

Nutrition Info per Serving

- Calories: 400
- Protein: 30g
- Carbohydrates: 30g
- Fat: 16g
- Fiber: 2g

Serves

- 4

Cooking Time

- 30 minutes

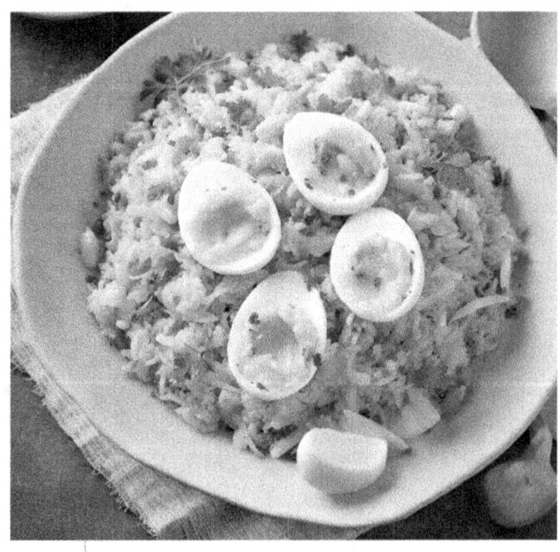

5. Sea Bass en Papillote

Ingredients

- 4 sea bass fillets
- 1 lemon, thinly sliced
- 1 zucchini, thinly sliced
- 1 red bell pepper, thinly sliced
- 2 tablespoons olive oil
- 1 tablespoon garlic-infused oil
- 1 teaspoon dried thyme
- 4 sheets of parchment paper

Instructions

1. Preheat your oven to 375°F (190°C).
2. Place each sea bass fillet on a sheet of parchment paper.
3. Top each fillet with lemon slices, zucchini, and red bell pepper.
4. Drizzle olive oil and garlic-infused oil over the fish and vegetables.
5. Sprinkle dried thyme over each fillet.
6. Fold the parchment paper over the fish and vegetables, sealing the edges to create a packet.
7. Place the packets on a baking sheet and bake for 20-25 minutes until the fish is cooked through.
8. Serve immediately.

Nutrition Info per Serving

- Calories: 250
- Protein: 30g
- Carbohydrates: 5g
- Fat: 12g
- Fiber: 2g

Serves

- 4

Cooking Time

- 30 minutes

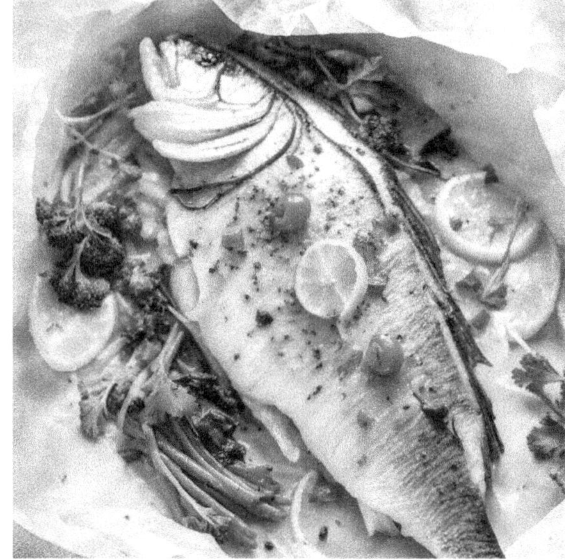

6. Shrimp and Grits

Ingredients

- 1 pound shrimp, peeled and deveined
- 1 cup gluten-free grits
- 4 cups water
- 1/2 cup lactose-free cheddar cheese, shredded
- 2 tablespoons garlic-infused oil
- 2 tablespoons olive oil
- 1 teaspoon smoked paprika
- 1/4 cup green onions, chopped (green parts only)
- 1 tablespoon lemon juice

Instructions

1. In a large pot, bring water to a boil. Add the grits and cook according to package instructions until creamy.
2. Stir in the shredded cheddar cheese and set aside.
3. In a large skillet, heat olive oil over medium-high heat.
4. Add the shrimp, garlic-infused oil, and smoked paprika. Cook for 3-4 minutes until the shrimp are pink and cooked through.
5. Stir in the lemon juice and green onions.
6. Serve the shrimp over the creamy grits.

Nutrition Info per Serving

- Calories: 320
- Protein: 25g
- Carbohydrates: 28g
- Fat: 14g
- Fiber: 2g

Serves

- 4

Cooking Time

- 25 minutes

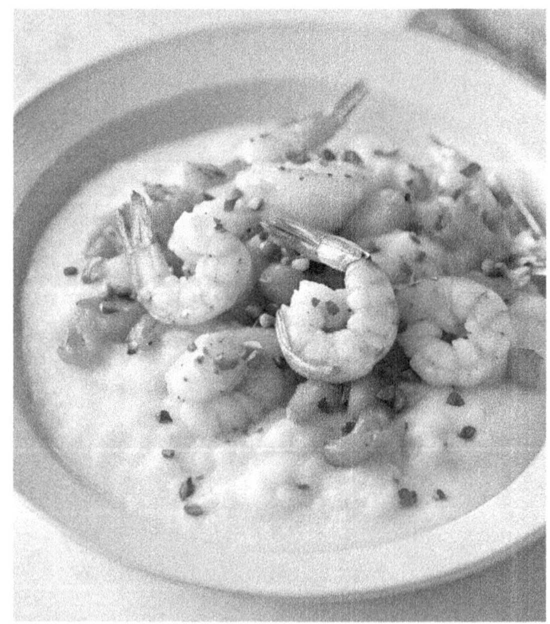

7. Crab Stuffed Flounder

Ingredients

- 4 flounder fillets
- 1 cup crab meat
- 1/4 cup gluten-free breadcrumbs
- 1/4 cup lactose-free cream cheese
- 1 tablespoon fresh parsley, chopped
- 1 tablespoon lemon juice
- 2 tablespoons olive oil

Instructions

1. Preheat your oven to 375°F (190°C).
2. In a bowl, mix together crab meat, gluten-free breadcrumbs, cream cheese, parsley, and lemon juice.
3. Place a spoonful of the crab mixture onto each flounder fillet and roll them up, securing with toothpicks if necessary.
4. Place the stuffed flounder in a baking dish and drizzle with olive oil.
5. Bake for 20-25 minutes until the fish is cooked through and the stuffing is golden brown.
6. Serve immediately.

Nutrition Info per Serving

- Calories: 280
- Protein: 25g
- Carbohydrates: 10g
- Fat: 16g
- Fiber: 1g

Serves

- 4

Cooking Time

- 30 minutes

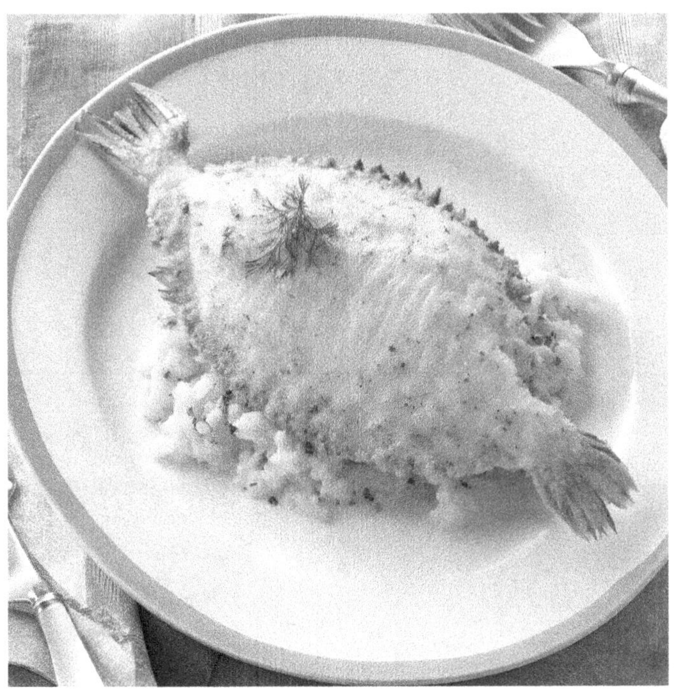

8. Halibut Steaks

Ingredients

- 4 halibut steaks
- 2 tablespoons olive oil
- 1 tablespoon garlic-infused oil
- 1 tablespoon lemon juice
- 1 teaspoon dried thyme
- 1/4 cup fresh parsley, chopped (for garnish)

Instructions

1. Preheat your grill or grill pan to medium-high heat.
2. In a small bowl, mix together olive oil, garlic-infused oil, lemon juice, and dried thyme.
3. Brush the halibut steaks with the mixture.
4. Grill the halibut steaks for 4-5 minutes on each side until cooked through.
5. Garnish with fresh parsley before serving.

Nutrition Info per Serving

- Calories: 290
- Protein: 35g
- Carbohydrates: 2g
- Fat: 16g
- Fiber: 1g

Serves

- 4

Cooking Time

- 15 minutes

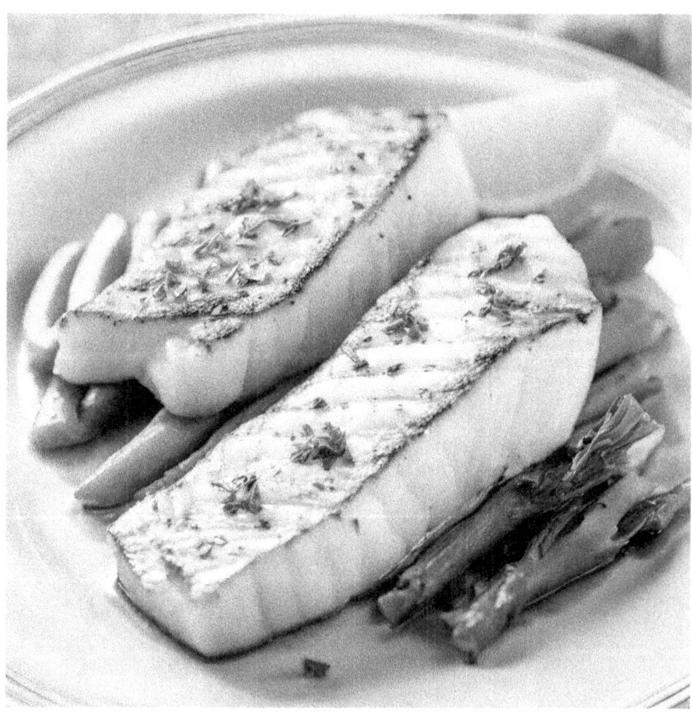

9. Lemon Baked Sole

Ingredients

- 4 sole fillets
- 2 tablespoons olive oil
- 1 lemon, thinly sliced
- 1 tablespoon garlic-infused oil
- 1 teaspoon dried oregano
- 1/4 cup fresh dill, chopped (for garnish)

Instructions

1. Preheat your oven to 375°F (190°C).
2. Place the sole fillets in a baking dish.
3. Drizzle olive oil and garlic-infused oil over the fillets.
4. Top with lemon slices and sprinkle with dried oregano.
5. Bake for 15-20 minutes until the fish is cooked through.
6. Garnish with fresh dill before serving.

Nutrition Info per Serving

- Calories: 220
- Protein: 28g
- Carbohydrates: 3g
- Fat: 10g
- Fiber: 1g

Serves

- 4

Cooking Time

- 20 minutes

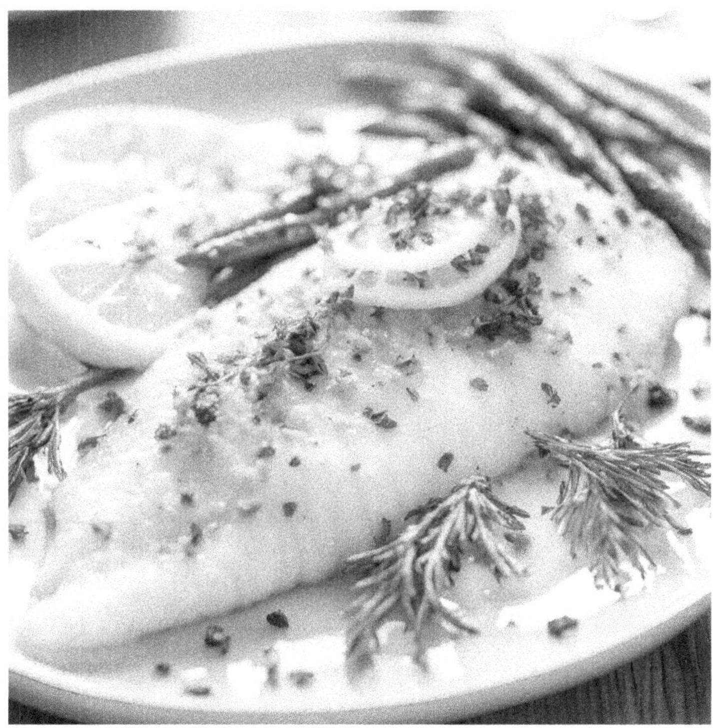

10. Pesto Shrimp Pasta

Ingredients

- 1 pound shrimp, peeled and deveined
- 8 ounces gluten-free pasta
- 1 cup fresh basil leaves
- 1/4 cup pine nuts
- 1/4 cup Parmesan cheese, grated
- 1/4 cup olive oil
- 1 tablespoon lemon juice
- 1 garlic clove, minced
- 1/2 cup cherry tomatoes, halved

Instructions

1. Cook the gluten-free pasta according to package instructions. Drain and set aside.
2. In a food processor, combine basil leaves, pine nuts, Parmesan cheese, olive oil, lemon juice, and minced garlic. Blend until smooth to make the pesto.
3. In a large skillet, heat 1 tablespoon of olive oil over medium-high heat. Add the shrimp and cook for 3-4 minutes until pink and cooked through.
4. Add the cooked pasta and pesto to the skillet with the shrimp. Toss to combine and heat through.
5. Stir in the cherry tomatoes and cook for an additional 1-2 minutes.
6. Serve immediately.

Nutrition Info per Serving

- Calories: 450
- Protein: 30g
- Carbohydrates: 45g
- Fat: 18g
- Fiber: 4g

Serves

- 4

Cooking Time

- 20 minutes

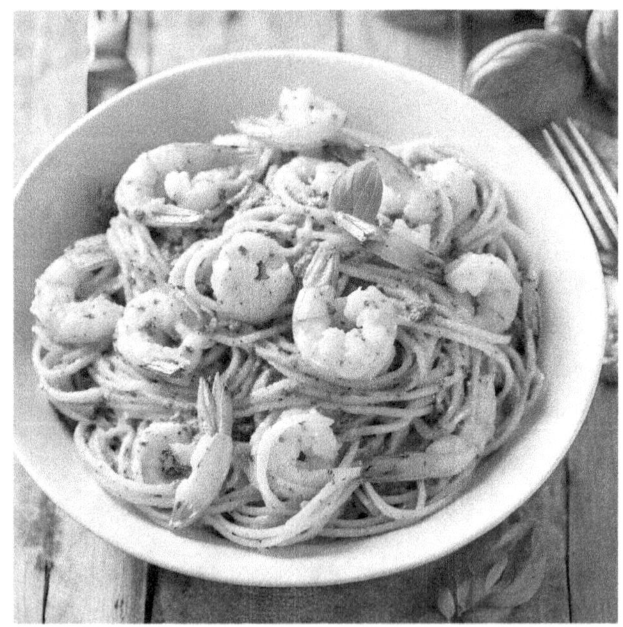

11. Salmon and Spinach Quiche

Ingredients

- 1 gluten-free pie crust
- 1 pound fresh salmon, cooked and flaked
- 1 cup fresh spinach, chopped
- 4 large eggs
- 1 cup lactose-free milk
- 1/2 cup lactose-free cheese, shredded
- 1 tablespoon garlic-infused oil
- 1 teaspoon dried dill

Instructions

1. Preheat your oven to 375°F (190°C).
2. Place the gluten-free pie crust in a pie dish.
3. Spread the flaked salmon and chopped spinach evenly in the pie crust.
4. In a bowl, whisk together eggs, lactose-free milk, shredded cheese, garlic-infused oil, and dried dill.
5. Pour the egg mixture over the salmon and spinach.
6. Bake for 30-35 minutes until the quiche is set and golden brown.
7. Let the quiche cool for a few minutes before slicing and serving.

Nutrition Info per Serving

- Calories: 350
- Protein: 28g
- Carbohydrates: 15g
- Fat: 20g
- Fiber: 2g

Serves

- 6

Cooking Time

- 40 minutes

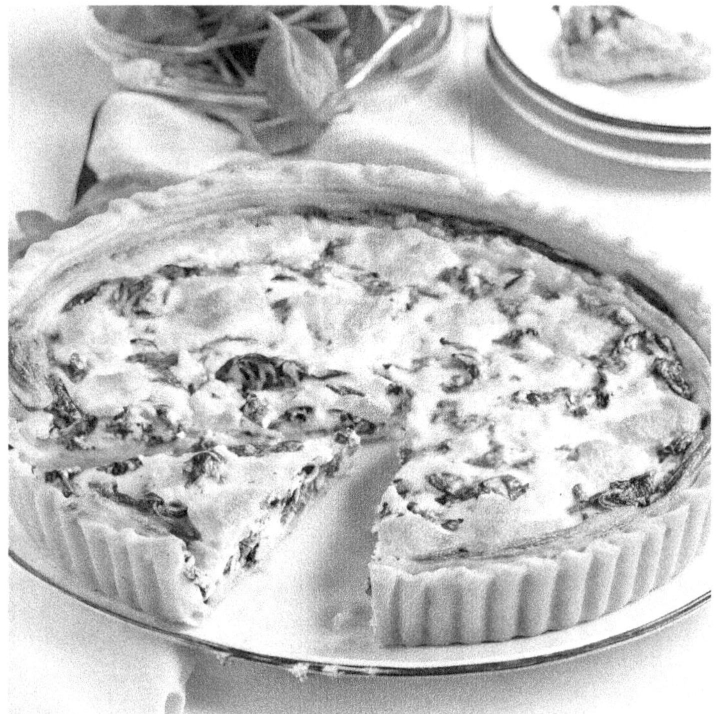

12. Anchovies Wrapped in Greens

Ingredients

- 1 can anchovies, drained
- 8 large Swiss chard or collard green leaves
- 2 tablespoons olive oil
- 1 tablespoon lemon juice
- 1 teaspoon garlic-infused oil

Instructions

1. Preheat your oven to 375°F (190°C).
2. Blanch the Swiss chard or collard green leaves in boiling water for 1-2 minutes until just tender. Drain and pat dry.
3. Place a few anchovies in the center of each leaf and roll up, tucking in the sides.
4. Place the wrapped anchovies in a baking dish.
5. In a small bowl, mix together olive oil, lemon juice, and garlic-infused oil.
6. Drizzle the mixture over the wrapped anchovies.
7. Bake for 15-20 minutes until heated through.
8. Serve immediately.

Nutrition Info per Serving

- Calories: 150
- Protein: 10g
- Carbohydrates: 2g
- Fat: 12g
- Fiber: 1g

Serves

- 4

Cooking Time

- 25 minutes

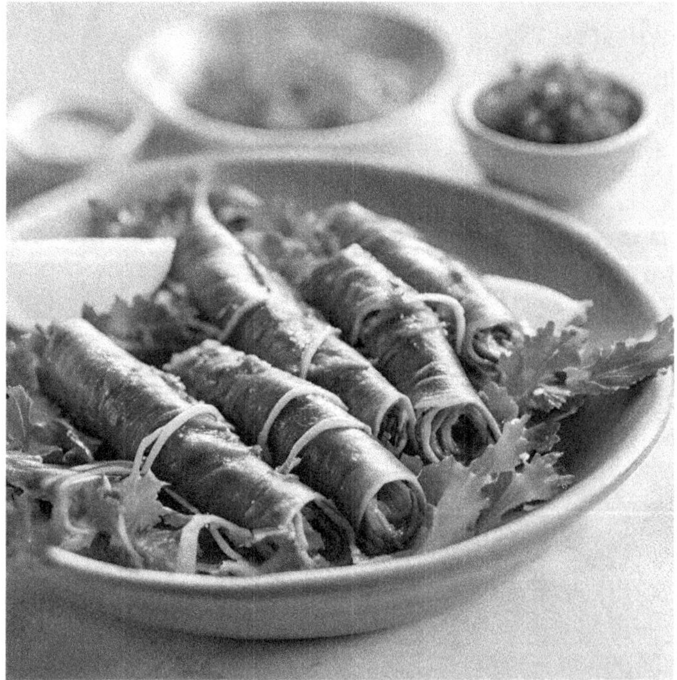

13. Seared Scallops

Ingredients

- 1 pound scallops, patted dry
- 2 tablespoons olive oil
- 1 tablespoon garlic-infused oil
- 1 tablespoon lemon juice
- 1 teaspoon dried thyme
- 1 tablespoon fresh parsley, chopped (for garnish)

Instructions

1. Heat olive oil in a large skillet over medium-high heat.
2. Add the scallops to the skillet and cook for 2-3 minutes on each side until they are golden brown and cooked through.
3. Remove the scallops from the skillet and set aside.
4. In the same skillet, add garlic-infused oil, lemon juice, and dried thyme. Cook for 1 minute until fragrant.
5. Return the scallops to the skillet and toss to coat with the sauce.
6. Garnish with fresh parsley before serving.

Nutrition Info per Serving

- Calories: 250
- Protein: 25g
- Carbohydrates: 3g
- Fat: 14g
- Fiber: 1g

Serves

- 4

Cooking Time

- 15 minutes

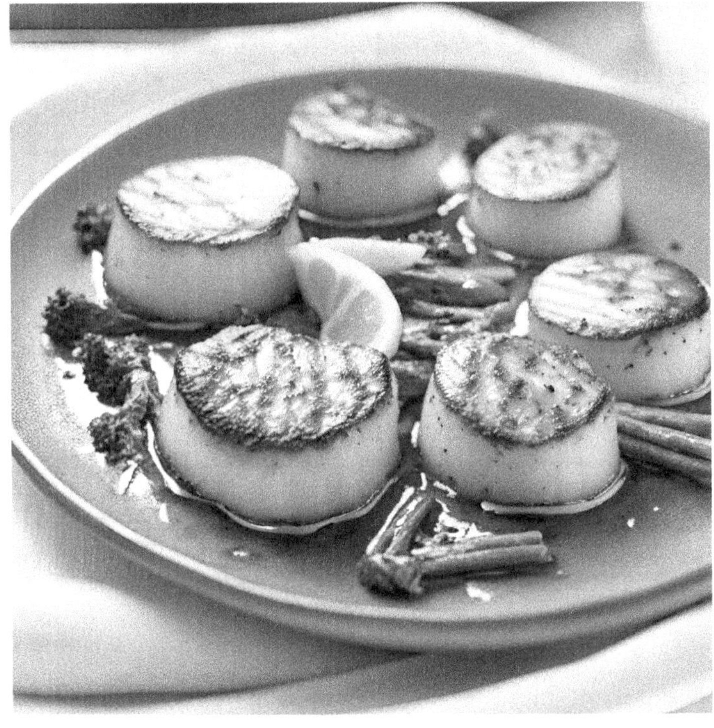

14. Grilled Swordfish

Ingredients

- 4 swordfish steaks
- 2 tablespoons olive oil
- 1 tablespoon lemon juice
- 1 tablespoon garlic-infused oil
- 1 teaspoon dried oregano
- 1/4 cup fresh basil, chopped (for garnish)

Instructions

1. Preheat your grill or grill pan to medium-high heat.
2. In a small bowl, mix together olive oil, lemon juice, garlic-infused oil, and dried oregano.
3. Brush the swordfish steaks with the mixture.
4. Grill the swordfish steaks for 4-5 minutes on each side until cooked through.
5. Garnish with fresh basil before serving.

Nutrition Info per Serving

- Calories: 300
- Protein: 35g
- Carbohydrates: 2g
- Fat: 16g
- Fiber: 1g

Serves

- 4

Cooking Time

- 15 minutes

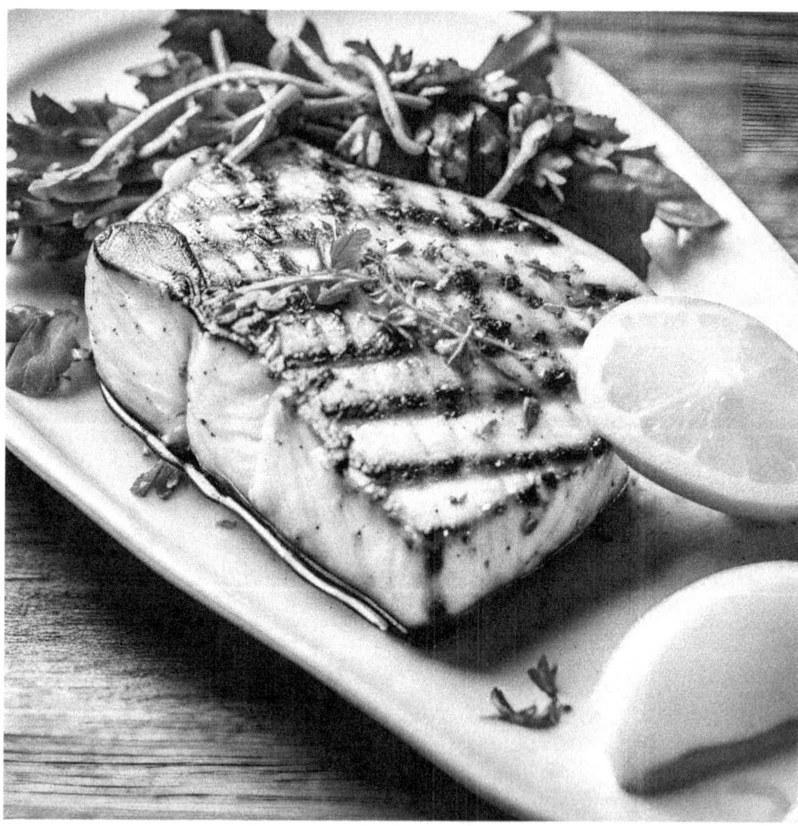

15. Baked Haddock

Ingredients

- 4 haddock fillets
- 2 tablespoons olive oil
- 1 tablespoon lemon juice
- 1 tablespoon garlic-infused oil
- 1 teaspoon dried thyme
- 1/4 cup gluten-free breadcrumbs
- 1 tablespoon fresh parsley, chopped (for garnish)

Instructions

1. Preheat your oven to 375°F (190°C).
2. Place the haddock fillets in a baking dish.
3. In a small bowl, mix together olive oil, lemon juice, garlic-infused oil, and dried thyme.
4. Brush the mixture over the haddock fillets.
5. Sprinkle gluten-free breadcrumbs evenly over the fillets.
6. Bake for 20-25 minutes until the fish is cooked through and the topping is golden brown.
7. Garnish with fresh parsley before serving.

Nutrition Info per Serving

- Calories: 240
- Protein: 28g
- Carbohydrates: 10g
- Fat: 10g
- Fiber: 2g

Serves

- 4

Cooking Time

- 30 minutes

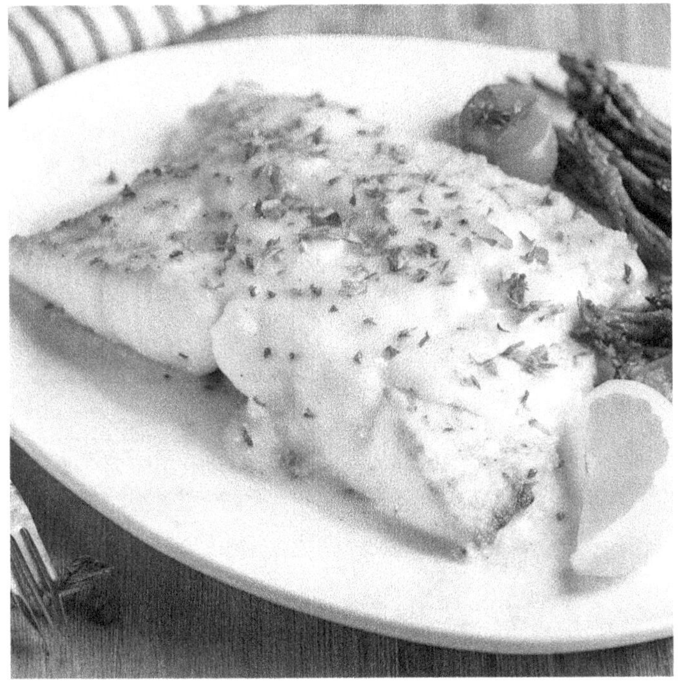

16. Pan-Fried Tilapia

Ingredients

- 4 tilapia fillets
- 2 tablespoons olive oil
- 1 tablespoon garlic-infused oil
- 1 teaspoon paprika
- 1 teaspoon dried oregano
- 1 tablespoon lemon juice

Instructions

1. Heat olive oil in a large skillet over medium-high heat.
2. In a small bowl, mix together garlic-infused oil, paprika, and dried oregano.
3. Brush the tilapia fillets with the oil and spice mixture.
4. Add the tilapia fillets to the skillet and cook for 3-4 minutes on each side until golden brown and cooked through.
5. Drizzle with lemon juice before serving.

Nutrition Info per Serving

- Calories: 220
- Protein: 28g
- Carbohydrates: 2g
- Fat: 12g
- Fiber: 1g

Serves

- 4

Cooking Time

- 15 minutes

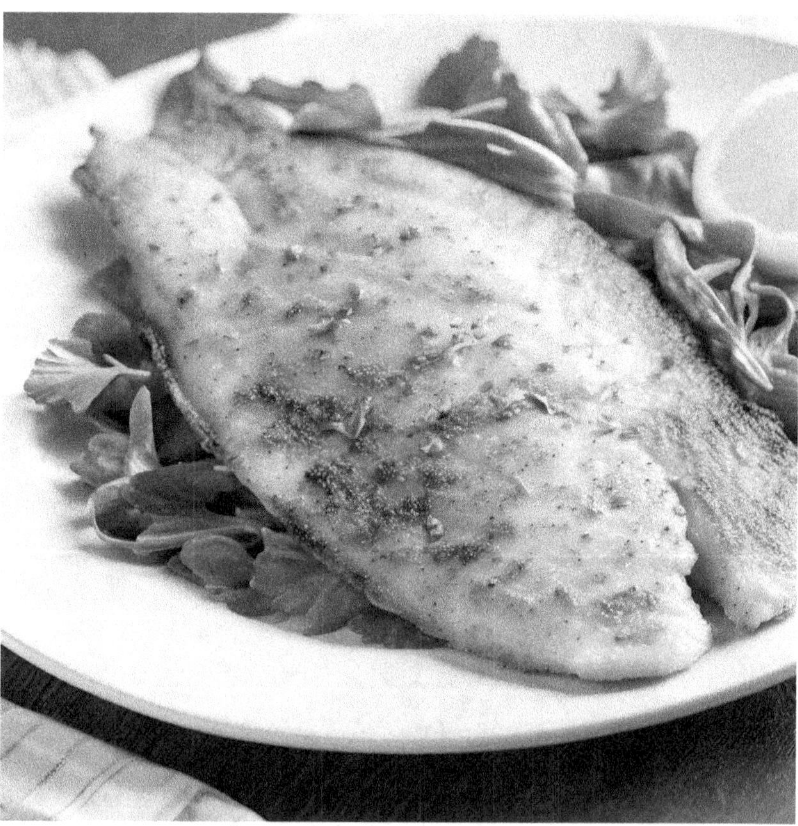

17. Canned Tuna Stir Fry

Ingredients

- 2 cans tuna in olive oil, drained
- 1 red bell pepper, sliced
- 1 green bell pepper, sliced
- 1 zucchini, sliced
- 2 tablespoons olive oil
- 1 tablespoon garlic-infused oil
- 2 tablespoons low-sodium tamari (gluten-free soy sauce)
- 1 tablespoon grated ginger

Instructions

1. Heat olive oil in a large skillet or wok over medium-high heat.
2. Add the garlic-infused oil and grated ginger. Cook for 1 minute until fragrant.
3. Add the red bell pepper, green bell pepper, and zucchini. Stir-fry for 3-4 minutes until the vegetables are tender-crisp.
4. Add the drained tuna and tamari. Stir-fry for another 2-3 minutes until heated through.
5. Serve immediately.

Nutrition Info per Serving

- Calories: 240
- Protein: 30g
- Carbohydrates: 8g
- Fat: 10g
- Fiber: 3g

Serves

- 4

Cooking Time

- 15 minutes

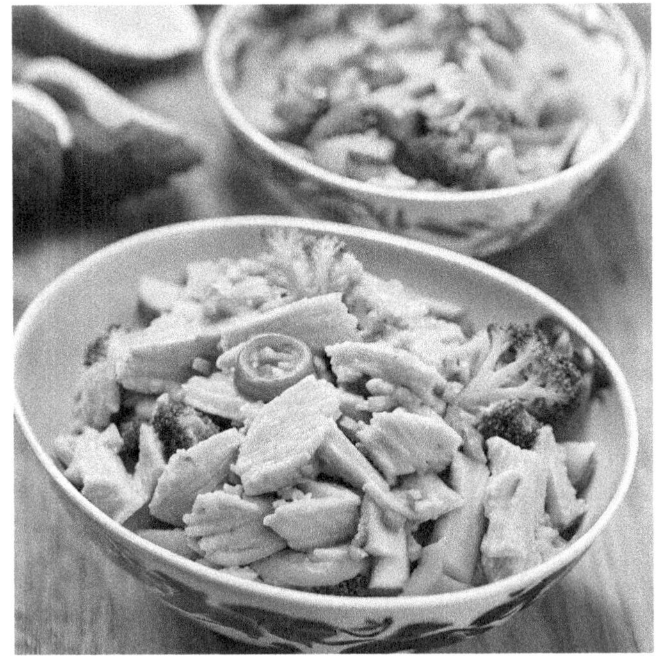

18. Smoked Herring

Ingredients

- 4 smoked herring fillets
- 1 tablespoon olive oil
- 1 tablespoon lemon juice
- 1 teaspoon garlic-infused oil
- 1/4 cup fresh parsley, chopped (for garnish)
- 1 lemon, cut into wedges (for serving)

Instructions

1. Preheat your oven to 350°F (175°C).
2. Place the smoked herring fillets on a baking sheet.
3. In a small bowl, mix together olive oil, lemon juice, and garlic-infused oil.
4. Brush the mixture over the herring fillets.
5. Bake for 10-12 minutes until heated through.
6. Garnish with fresh parsley and serve with lemon wedges.

Nutrition Info per Serving

- Calories: 200
- Protein: 22g
- Carbohydrates: 2g
- Fat: 12g
- Fiber: 1g

Serves

- 4

Cooking Time

- 15 minutes

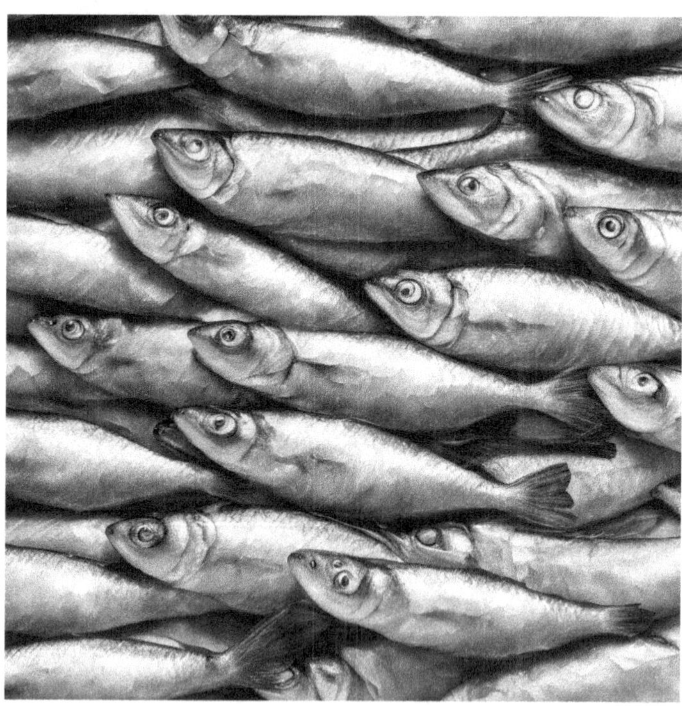

19. Sardine and Tomato Pasta

Ingredients

- 2 cans sardines in olive oil, drained
- 8 ounces gluten-free pasta
- 1 cup cherry tomatoes, halved
- 2 tablespoons olive oil
- 1 tablespoon garlic-infused oil
- 1 teaspoon dried oregano
- 1/4 cup fresh basil, chopped
- 1 tablespoon lemon juice

Instructions

1. Cook the gluten-free pasta according to package instructions. Drain and set aside.
2. In a large skillet, heat olive oil over medium heat. Add garlic-infused oil and cook for 1 minute until fragrant.
3. Add the cherry tomatoes and dried oregano. Cook for 3-4 minutes until the tomatoes start to soften.
4. Add the drained sardines and cook for another 2-3 minutes until heated through.
5. Toss the cooked pasta with the sardine and tomato mixture.
6. Stir in the fresh basil and lemon juice.
7. Serve immediately.

Nutrition Info per Serving

- Calories: 350
- Protein: 25g
- Carbohydrates: 35g
- Fat: 14g
- Fiber: 4g

Serves

- 4

Cooking Time

- 20 minutes

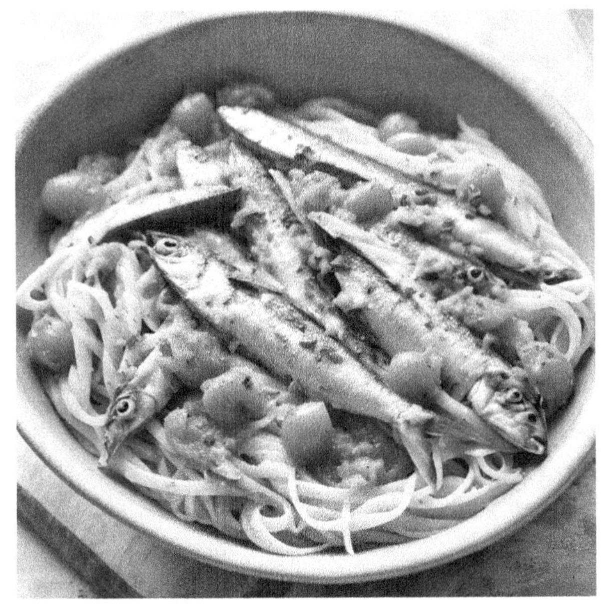

20. Salmon Burgers

Ingredients

- 1 pound fresh salmon, skin removed and finely chopped
- 1/4 cup gluten-free breadcrumbs
- 1 egg, beaten
- 2 tablespoons fresh parsley, chopped
- 1 tablespoon Dijon mustard
- 1 tablespoon lemon juice
- 1 tablespoon garlic-infused oil
- 2 tablespoons olive oil (for cooking)
- 4 gluten-free burger buns
- Lettuce, tomato, and avocado for serving

Instructions

1. In a large bowl, combine the chopped salmon, gluten-free breadcrumbs, beaten egg, parsley, Dijon mustard, lemon juice, and garlic-infused oil. Mix until well combined.
2. Form the mixture into 4 equal patties.
3. Heat olive oil in a large skillet over medium-high heat.
4. Cook the salmon patties for 4-5 minutes on each side until golden brown and cooked through.
5. Serve the salmon burgers on gluten-free buns with lettuce, tomato, and avocado.

Nutrition Info per Serving

- Calories: 350
- Protein: 28g
- Carbohydrates: 20g
- Fat: 18g
- Fiber: 3g

Serves

- 4

Cooking Time

- 20 minutes

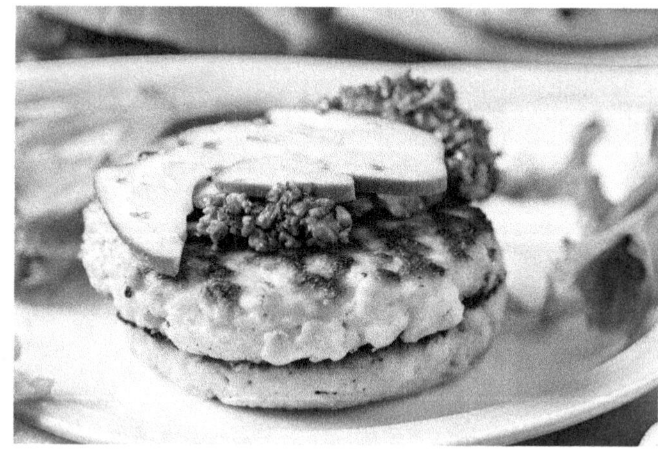

21. Grilled Mackerel

Ingredients

- 4 mackerel fillets
- 2 tablespoons olive oil
- 1 tablespoon lemon juice
- 1 teaspoon garlic-infused oil
- 1 teaspoon dried oregano
- 1/4 cup fresh parsley, chopped (for garnish)

Instructions

1. Preheat your grill or grill pan to medium-high heat.
2. In a small bowl, mix together olive oil, lemon juice, garlic-infused oil, and dried oregano.
3. Brush the mackerel fillets with the mixture.
4. Grill the mackerel fillets for 4-5 minutes on each side until cooked through.
5. Garnish with fresh parsley before serving.

Nutrition Info per Serving

- Calories: 280
- Protein: 25g
- Carbohydrates: 2g
- Fat: 18g
- Fiber: 1g

Serves

- 4

Cooking Time

- 15 minutes

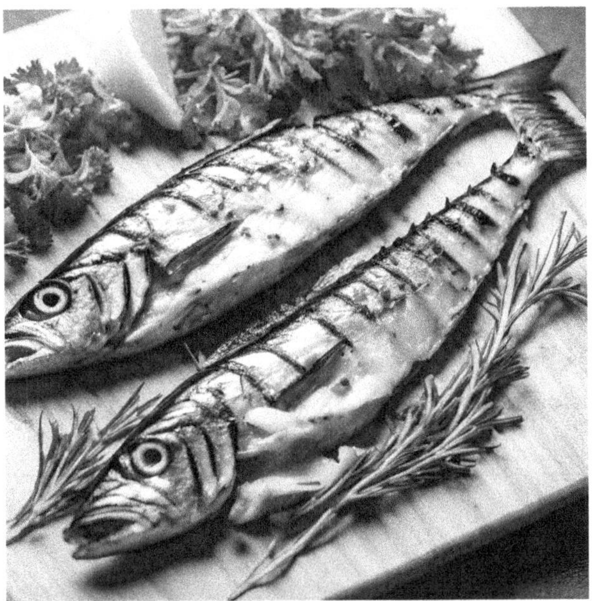

22. Clam Chowder

Ingredients

- 2 cups clams, chopped (fresh or canned)
- 4 cups low-sodium chicken broth
- 1 cup lactose-free milk
- 2 potatoes, diced
- 1 onion, diced
- 2 celery stalks, diced
- 2 tablespoons olive oil
- 1 tablespoon garlic-infused oil
- 1 teaspoon dried thyme
- 1 bay leaf
- 1/4 cup fresh parsley, chopped (for garnish)

Instructions

1. In a large pot, heat olive oil over medium heat.
2. Add the diced onion and celery. Cook until softened, about 5 minutes.
3. Stir in the garlic-infused oil, dried thyme, and bay leaf. Cook for 1 minute.
4. Add the diced potatoes, chicken broth, and clams to the pot. Bring to a boil, then reduce heat and simmer for 15-20 minutes until the potatoes are tender.
5. Stir in the lactose-free milk and cook for another 5 minutes until heated through.
6. Remove the bay leaf before serving.
7. Garnish with fresh parsley before serving.

Nutrition Info per Serving

- Calories: 250
- Protein: 20g
- Carbohydrates: 25g
- Fat: 8g
- Fiber: 3g

Serves

- 4

Cooking Time

- 30 minutes

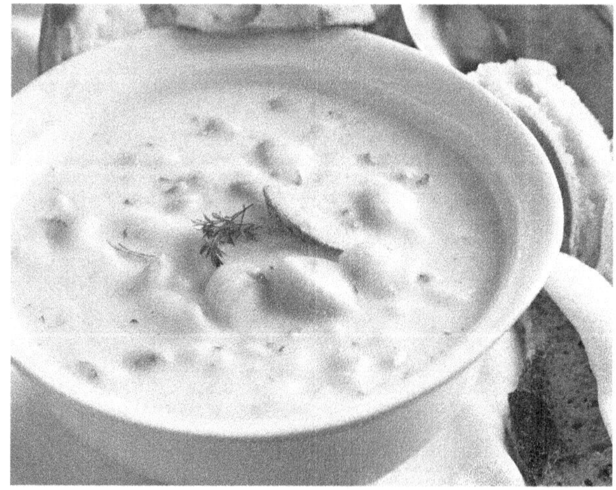

23. Baked Trout

Ingredients

- 4 trout fillets
- 2 tablespoons olive oil
- 1 lemon, thinly sliced
- 1 tablespoon garlic-infused oil
- 1 teaspoon dried thyme
- 1/4 cup fresh dill, chopped (for garnish)

Instructions

1. Preheat your oven to 375°F (190°C).
2. Place the trout fillets in a baking dish.
3. In a small bowl, mix together olive oil, garlic-infused oil, and dried thyme.
4. Brush the mixture over the trout fillets.
5. Top each fillet with lemon slices.
6. Bake for 20-25 minutes until the fish is cooked through.
7. Garnish with fresh dill before serving.

Nutrition Info per Serving

- Calories: 240
- Protein: 28g
- Carbohydrates: 3g
- Fat: 12g
- Fiber: 1g

Serves

- 4

Cooking Time

- 30 minutes

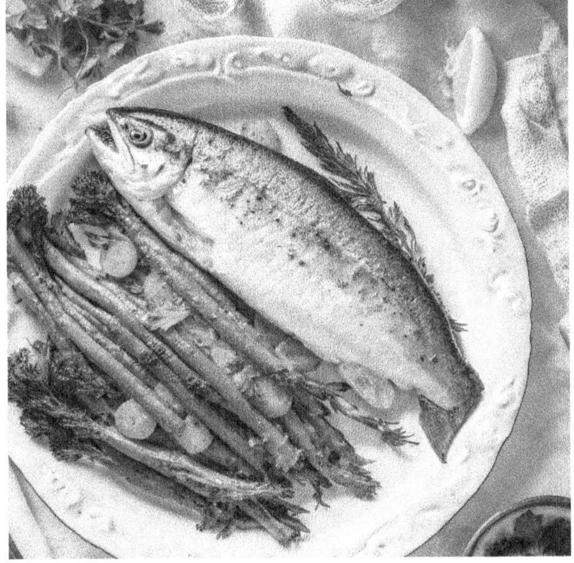

24. Oyster Mushroom Ceviche
Ingredients

- 1 pound oyster mushrooms, thinly sliced
- 1/2 cup lime juice
- 1/4 cup lemon juice
- 1 tablespoon garlic-infused oil
- 1 red bell pepper, finely diced
- 1/2 cucumber, finely diced
- 1/4 cup fresh cilantro, chopped
- 1 avocado, diced

Instructions

1. In a large bowl, combine the sliced oyster mushrooms, lime juice, lemon juice, and garlic-infused oil. Mix well and let marinate in the refrigerator for at least 30 minutes.
2. Add the diced red bell pepper, cucumber, and fresh cilantro to the bowl. Toss to combine.
3. Gently fold in the diced avocado.
4. Serve immediately.

Nutrition Info per Serving

- Calories: 180
- Protein: 5g
- Carbohydrates: 15g
- Fat: 12g
- Fiber: 6g

Serves

- 4

Cooking Time

- 40 minutes (including marinating time)

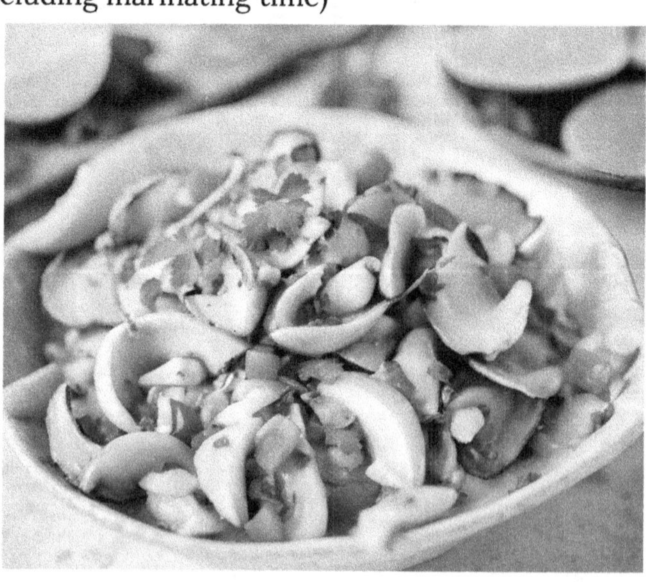

25. Garlic-Infused Olive Oil Scallops

Ingredients

- 1 pound scallops, patted dry
- 2 tablespoons garlic-infused olive oil
- 1 tablespoon lemon juice
- 1 teaspoon dried thyme
- 1 tablespoon fresh parsley, chopped (for garnish)

Instructions

1. Heat the garlic-infused olive oil in a large skillet over medium-high heat.
2. Add the scallops to the skillet and cook for 2-3 minutes on each side until they are golden brown and cooked through.
3. Remove the scallops from the skillet and set aside.
4. In the same skillet, add the lemon juice and dried thyme. Cook for 1 minute until fragrant.
5. Return the scallops to the skillet and toss to coat with the sauce.
6. Garnish with fresh parsley before serving.

Nutrition Info per Serving

- Calories: 240
- Protein: 24g
- Carbohydrates: 3g
- Fat: 14g
- Fiber: 1g

Serves

- 4

Cooking Time

- 15 minutes

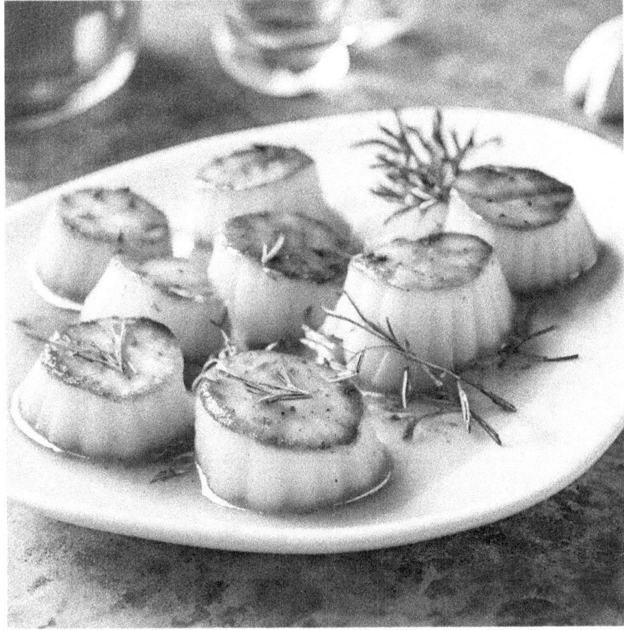

Soup and Stew Recipes

1. Vegetable and Lentil Stew

Ingredients

- 1 cup green or brown lentils, rinsed
- 1 onion, diced
- 2 carrots, sliced
- 2 celery stalks, sliced
- 1 red bell pepper, diced
- 2 cups diced tomatoes (canned, no added salt)
- 4 cups vegetable broth (low sodium)
- 2 tablespoons olive oil
- 1 tablespoon garlic-infused oil
- 1 teaspoon dried thyme
- 1 teaspoon ground cumin
- 1/2 teaspoon smoked paprika
- 1/4 cup fresh parsley, chopped (for garnish)

Instructions

1. In a large pot, heat olive oil over medium heat.
2. Add the diced onion, carrots, and celery. Cook until softened, about 5 minutes.
3. Stir in the garlic-infused oil, ground cumin, and smoked paprika. Cook for another 1-2 minutes.
4. Add the diced red bell pepper, diced tomatoes, lentils, and vegetable broth. Bring to a boil.
5. Reduce heat and simmer for 30-35 minutes until the lentils are tender.
6. Garnish with fresh parsley before serving.

Nutrition Info per Serving

- Calories: 250
- Protein: 12g
- Carbohydrates: 40g
- Fat: 8g
- Fiber: 15g

Serves

- 4

Cooking Time

- 45 minutes

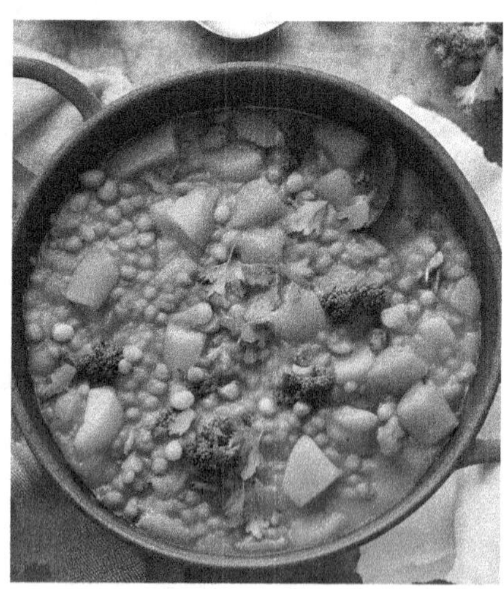

2. White Fish Stew

Ingredients

- 1 pound white fish fillets (such as cod or haddock), cut into chunks
- 1 onion, diced
- 2 carrots, sliced
- 1 fennel bulb, sliced
- 2 cups diced tomatoes (canned, no added salt)
- 4 cups fish or vegetable broth (low sodium)
- 2 tablespoons olive oil
- 1 tablespoon garlic-infused oil
- 1 teaspoon dried thyme
- 1/2 teaspoon saffron threads (optional)
- 1/4 cup fresh dill, chopped (for garnish)

Instructions

1. In a large pot, heat olive oil over medium heat.
2. Add the diced onion, carrots, and fennel. Cook until softened, about 5 minutes.
3. Stir in the garlic-infused oil and dried thyme. Cook for another 1-2 minutes.
4. Add the diced tomatoes and broth. Bring to a boil.
5. Reduce heat and simmer for 20 minutes.
6. Add the fish chunks and saffron threads (if using). Simmer for another 10 minutes until the fish is cooked through.
7. Garnish with fresh dill before serving.

Nutrition Info per Serving

- Calories: 220
- Protein: 28g
- Carbohydrates: 15g
- Fat: 8g
- Fiber: 4g

Serves

- 4

Cooking Time

- 40 minutes

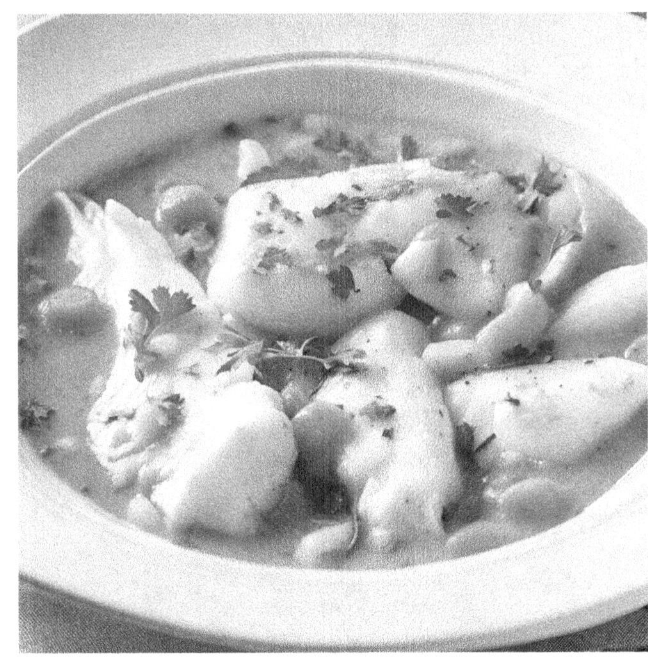

3. Broccoli Soup

Ingredients

- 4 cups broccoli florets
- 1 onion, diced
- 2 cups potatoes, peeled and diced
- 4 cups vegetable broth (low sodium)
- 1 cup lactose-free milk
- 2 tablespoons olive oil
- 1 tablespoon garlic-infused oil
- 1 teaspoon dried thyme
- 1/4 cup lactose-free cheddar cheese, shredded (optional)
- 1/4 cup fresh chives, chopped (for garnish)

Instructions

1. In a large pot, heat olive oil over medium heat.
2. Add the diced onion and cook until softened, about 5 minutes.
3. Stir in the garlic-infused oil and dried thyme. Cook for another 1-2 minutes.
4. Add the broccoli florets, potatoes, and vegetable broth. Bring to a boil.
5. Reduce heat and simmer for 20 minutes until the vegetables are tender.
6. Puree the soup using an immersion blender or in batches using a regular blender until smooth.
7. Stir in the lactose-free milk and heat through.
8. Optionally, stir in the shredded cheddar cheese until melted.
9. Garnish with fresh chives before serving.

Nutrition Info per Serving

- Calories: 200
- Protein: 8g
- Carbohydrates: 28g
- Fat: 8g
- Fiber: 6g

Serves

- 4

Cooking Time

- 30 minutes

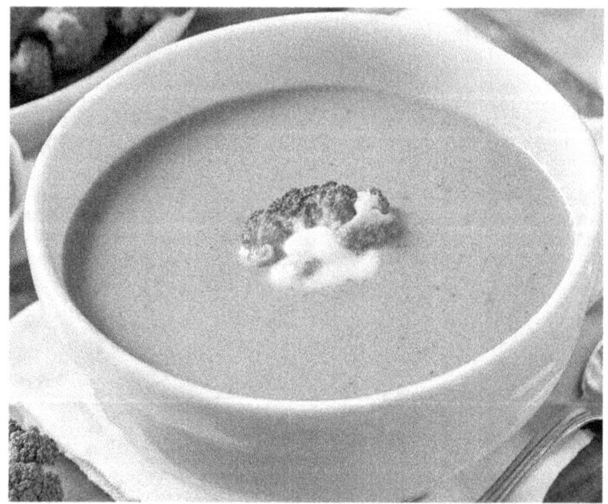

4. Irish Stew

Ingredients

- 1 pound lamb shoulder, cut into chunks
- 4 cups potatoes, peeled and diced
- 2 carrots, sliced
- 2 celery stalks, sliced
- 1 onion, diced
- 4 cups beef broth (low sodium)
- 2 tablespoons olive oil
- 1 tablespoon garlic-infused oil
- 1 teaspoon dried thyme
- 1 teaspoon dried rosemary
- 1/4 cup fresh parsley, chopped (for garnish)

Instructions

1. In a large pot or Dutch oven, heat olive oil over medium-high heat.
2. Add the lamb chunks and cook until browned on all sides, about 5-7 minutes. Remove the lamb and set aside.
3. In the same pot, add the diced onion, carrots, and celery. Cook until softened, about 5 minutes.
4. Stir in the garlic-infused oil, dried thyme, and dried rosemary. Cook for another 1-2 minutes.
5. Return the lamb to the pot and add the potatoes and beef broth. Bring to a boil.
6. Reduce heat and simmer for 1.5 to 2 hours until the lamb is tender.
7. Garnish with fresh parsley before serving.

Nutrition Info per Serving

- Calories: 350
- Protein: 25g
- Carbohydrates: 35g
- Fat: 12g
- Fiber: 6g

Serves

- 4

Cooking Time

- 2 hours 15 minutes

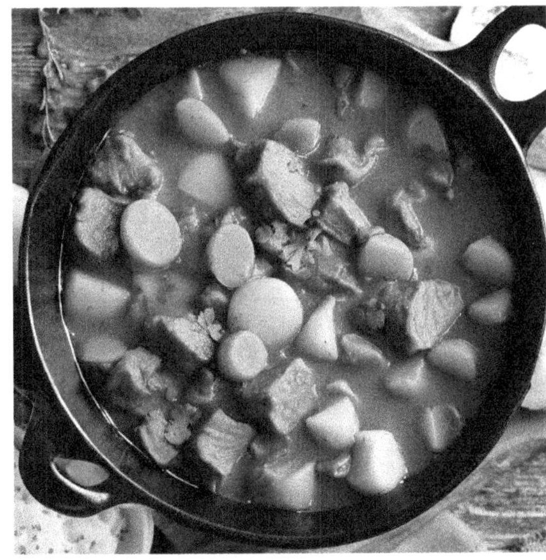

5. Spicy Chicken Stew

Ingredients

- 1 pound boneless, skinless chicken thighs, cut into chunks
- 1 onion, diced
- 2 carrots, sliced
- 2 celery stalks, sliced
- 1 red bell pepper, diced
- 4 cups chicken broth (low sodium)
- 1 can diced tomatoes (canned, no added salt)
- 2 tablespoons olive oil
- 1 tablespoon garlic-infused oil
- 1 tablespoon chili powder
- 1 teaspoon cumin
- 1/2 teaspoon cayenne pepper
- 1/4 cup fresh cilantro, chopped (for garnish)

Instructions

1. In a large pot, heat olive oil over medium-high heat.
2. Add the chicken chunks and cook until browned on all sides, about 5-7 minutes. Remove the chicken and set aside.
3. In the same pot, add the diced onion, carrots, and celery. Cook until softened, about 5 minutes.
4. Stir in the garlic-infused oil, chili powder, cumin, and cayenne pepper. Cook for another 1-2 minutes.
5. Add the diced red bell pepper, chicken broth, and diced tomatoes. Bring to a boil.
6. Return the chicken to the pot. Reduce heat and simmer for 30 minutes until the vegetables are tender and the chicken is cooked through.
7. Garnish with fresh cilantro before serving.

Nutrition Info per Serving

- Calories: 300
- Protein: 25g
- Carbohydrates: 20g
- Fat: 12g
- Fiber: 4g

Serves

- 4

Cooking Time

- 45 minutes

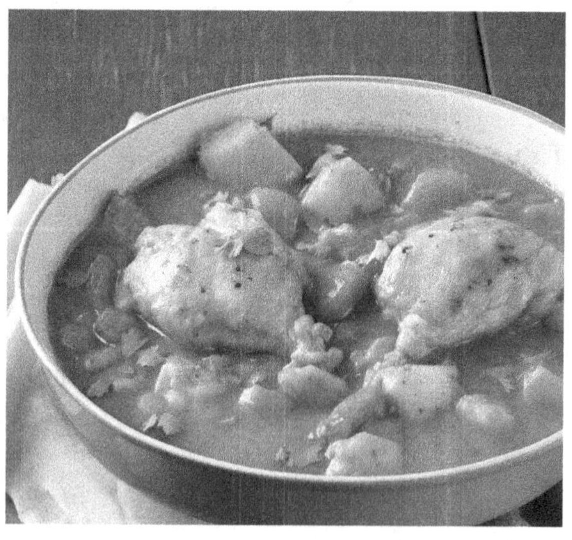

6. Sweet Potato and Ginger Soup

Ingredients

- 2 large sweet potatoes, peeled and diced
- 1 onion, diced
- 1 tablespoon ginger, grated
- 4 cups vegetable broth (low sodium)
- 1 cup coconut milk (canned)
- 2 tablespoons olive oil
- 1 tablespoon garlic-infused oil
- 1/2 teaspoon ground cumin
- 1/4 teaspoon ground cinnamon
- 1/4 cup fresh cilantro, chopped (for garnish)

Instructions

1. In a large pot, heat olive oil over medium heat.
2. Add the diced onion and cook until softened, about 5 minutes.
3. Stir in the garlic-infused oil, grated ginger, ground cumin, and ground cinnamon. Cook for another 1-2 minutes.
4. Add the diced sweet potatoes and vegetable broth. Bring to a boil.
5. Reduce heat and simmer for 20-25 minutes until the sweet potatoes are tender.
6. Puree the soup using an immersion blender or in batches using a regular blender until smooth.
7. Stir in the coconut milk and heat through.
8. Garnish with fresh cilantro before serving.

Nutrition Info per Serving

- Calories: 250
- Protein: 4g
- Carbohydrates: 35g
- Fat: 10g
- Fiber: 6g

Serves

- 4

Cooking Time

- 35 minutes

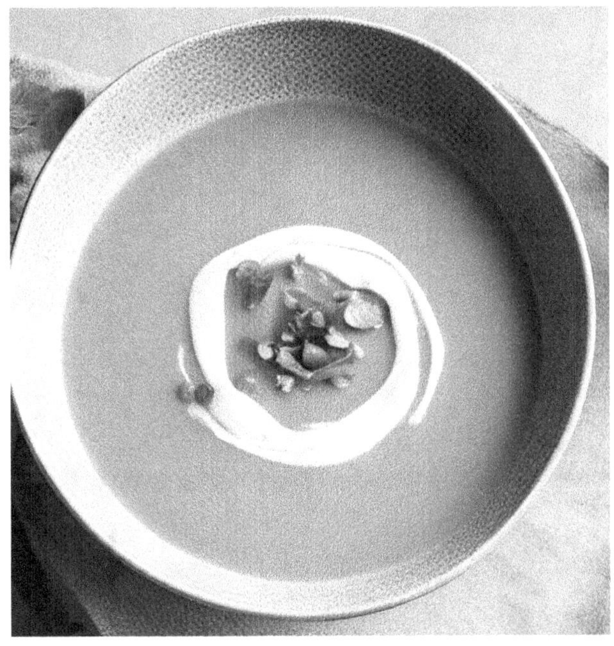

7. Leek and Potato Soup

Ingredients

- 4 cups leeks, sliced (white and light green parts only)
- 2 cups potatoes, peeled and diced
- 1 onion, diced
- 4 cups chicken broth (low sodium)
- 1 cup lactose-free milk
- 2 tablespoons olive oil
- 1 tablespoon garlic-infused oil
- 1 teaspoon dried thyme
- 1/4 cup fresh chives, chopped (for garnish)

Instructions

1. In a large pot, heat olive oil over medium heat.
2. Add the sliced leeks and diced onion. Cook until softened, about 5 minutes.
3. Stir in the garlic-infused oil and dried thyme. Cook for another 1-2 minutes.
4. Add the diced potatoes and chicken broth. Bring to a boil.
5. Reduce heat and simmer for 20-25 minutes until the potatoes are tender.
6. Puree the soup using an immersion blender or in batches using a regular blender until smooth.
7. Stir in the lactose-free milk and heat through.
8. Garnish with fresh chives before serving.

Nutrition Info per Serving

- Calories: 220
- Protein: 6g
- Carbohydrates: 32g
- Fat: 8g
- Fiber: 5g

Serves

- 4

Cooking Time

- 35 minutes

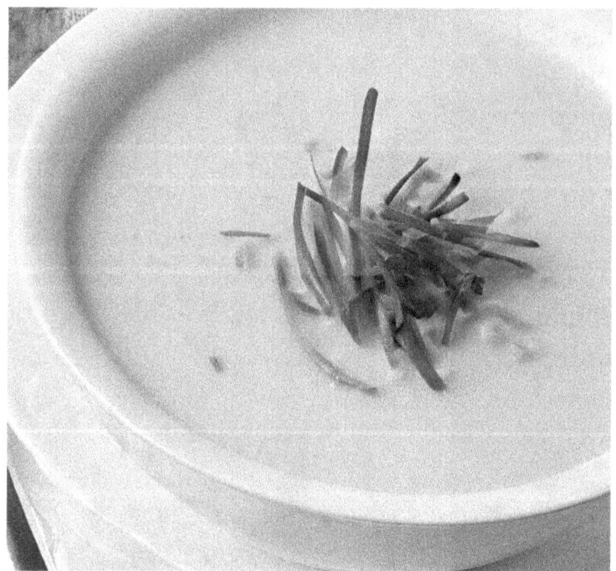

8. Sauerkraut Soup

Ingredients

- 2 cups sauerkraut, drained
- 1 pound smoked sausage, sliced
- 1 onion, diced
- 2 carrots, sliced
- 2 celery stalks, sliced
- 4 cups chicken broth (low sodium)
- 2 tablespoons olive oil
- 1 tablespoon garlic-infused oil
- 1 teaspoon caraway seeds
- 1/2 teaspoon smoked paprika
- 1/4 cup fresh parsley, chopped (for garnish)

Instructions

1. In a large pot, heat olive oil over medium heat.
2. Add the diced onion, carrots, and celery. Cook until softened, about 5 minutes.
3. Stir in the garlic-infused oil, caraway seeds, and smoked paprika. Cook for another 1-2 minutes.
4. Add the sliced smoked sausage, sauerkraut, and chicken broth. Bring to a boil.
5. Reduce heat and simmer for 25-30 minutes until the vegetables are tender and the flavors are well combined.
6. Garnish with fresh parsley before serving.

Nutrition Info per Serving

- Calories: 280
- Protein: 14g
- Carbohydrates: 20g
- Fat: 16g
- Fiber: 5g

Serves

- 4

Cooking Time

- 40 minutes

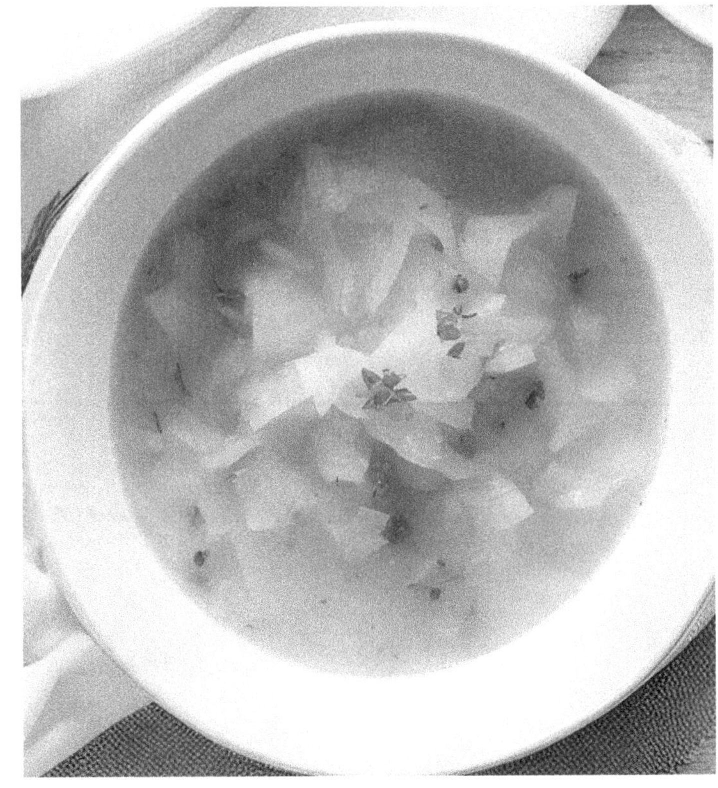

9. Chicken Tortilla Soup

Ingredients

- 1 pound boneless, skinless chicken breasts, shredded
- 1 onion, diced
- 1 red bell pepper, diced
- 1 can diced tomatoes (canned, no added salt)
- 4 cups chicken broth (low sodium)
- 1 tablespoon garlic-infused oil
- 1 teaspoon ground cumin
- 1 teaspoon chili powder
- 4 corn tortillas, cut into strips and baked until crispy
- 1/4 cup fresh cilantro, chopped (for garnish)
- 1 avocado, diced (for garnish)
- 1 lime, cut into wedges (for serving)

Instructions

1. In a large pot, heat garlic-infused oil over medium heat.
2. Add the diced onion and red bell pepper. Cook until softened, about 5 minutes.
3. Stir in the ground cumin and chili powder. Cook for another 1-2 minutes.
4. Add the shredded chicken, diced tomatoes, and chicken broth. Bring to a boil.
5. Reduce heat and simmer for 20-25 minutes until the flavors are well combined.
6. Serve the soup topped with crispy tortilla strips, fresh cilantro, diced avocado, and lime wedges.

Nutrition Info per Serving

- Calories: 320
- Protein: 25g
- Carbohydrates: 25g
- Fat: 12g
- Fiber: 6g

Serves

- 4

Cooking Time

- 35 minutes

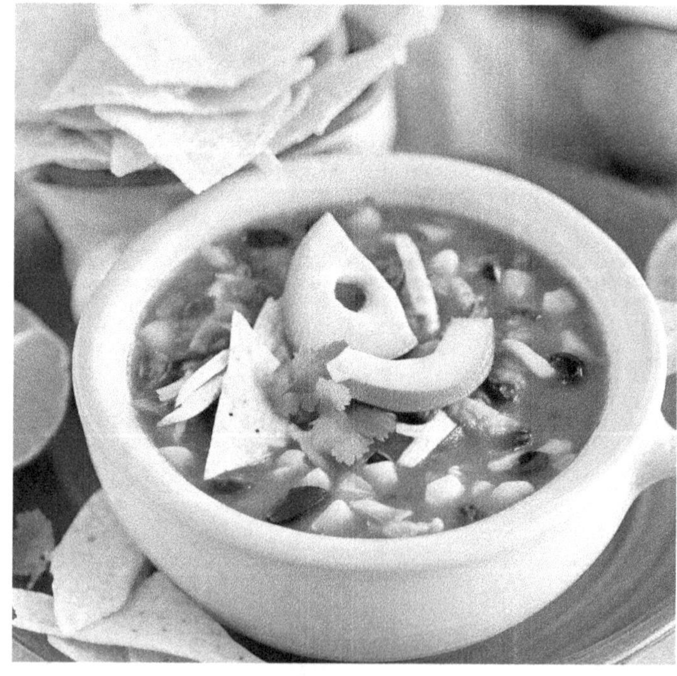

10. Cauliflower and Turmeric Soup

Ingredients

- 1 head cauliflower, cut into florets
- 1 onion, diced
- 1 tablespoon garlic-infused oil
- 4 cups vegetable broth (low sodium)
- 1 cup coconut milk (canned)
- 1 tablespoon olive oil
- 1 teaspoon ground turmeric
- 1/2 teaspoon ground cumin
- 1/4 teaspoon ground ginger
- 1/4 cup fresh cilantro, chopped (for garnish)

Instructions

1. In a large pot, heat olive oil over medium heat.
2. Add the diced onion and cook until softened, about 5 minutes.
3. Stir in the garlic-infused oil, ground turmeric, ground cumin, and ground ginger. Cook for another 1-2 minutes.
4. Add the cauliflower florets and vegetable broth. Bring to a boil.
5. Reduce heat and simmer for 20-25 minutes until the cauliflower is tender.
6. Puree the soup using an immersion blender or in batches using a regular blender until smooth.
7. Stir in the coconut milk and heat through.
8. Garnish with fresh cilantro before serving.

Nutrition Info per Serving

- Calories: 240
- Protein: 6g
- Carbohydrates: 20g
- Fat: 16g
- Fiber: 6g

Serves

- 4

Cooking Time

- 35 minutes

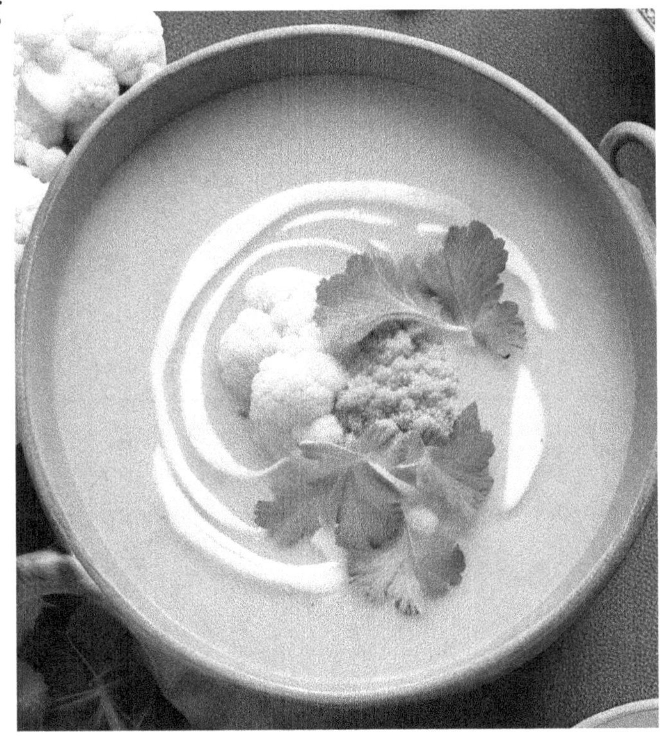

11. Quinoa Vegetable Stew

Ingredients

- 1 cup quinoa, rinsed
- 1 onion, diced
- 2 carrots, sliced
- 2 celery stalks, sliced
- 1 zucchini, diced
- 1 red bell pepper, diced
- 4 cups vegetable broth (low sodium)
- 1 can diced tomatoes (canned, no added salt)
- 2 tablespoons olive oil
- 1 tablespoon garlic-infused oil
- 1 teaspoon dried thyme
- 1 teaspoon ground cumin
- 1/4 cup fresh parsley, chopped (for garnish)

Instructions

1. In a large pot, heat olive oil over medium heat.
2. Add the diced onion, carrots, and celery. Cook until softened, about 5 minutes.
3. Stir in the garlic-infused oil, dried thyme, and ground cumin. Cook for another 1-2 minutes.
4. Add the diced zucchini, red bell pepper, quinoa, vegetable broth, and diced tomatoes. Bring to a boil.
5. Reduce heat and simmer for 20-25 minutes until the quinoa is cooked and the vegetables are tender.
6. Garnish with fresh parsley before serving.

Nutrition Info per Serving

- Calories: 300
- Protein: 8g
- Carbohydrates: 50g
- Fat: 10g
- Fiber: 8g

Serves

- 4

Cooking Time

- 35 minutes

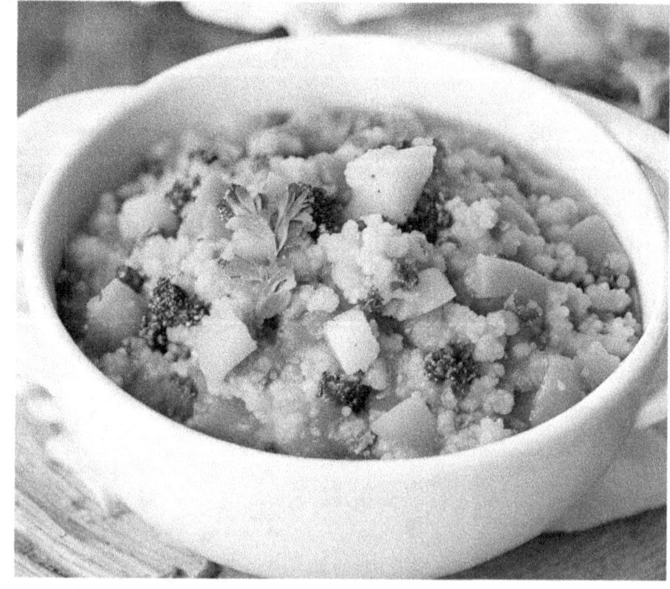

12. Zucchini Soup

Ingredients

- 4 cups zucchini, sliced
- 1 onion, diced
- 2 cups potatoes, peeled and diced
- 4 cups chicken broth (low sodium)
- 1 cup lactose-free milk
- 2 tablespoons olive oil
- 1 tablespoon garlic-infused oil
- 1 teaspoon dried thyme
- 1/4 cup fresh chives, chopped (for garnish)

Instructions

1. In a large pot, heat olive oil over medium heat.
2. Add the diced onion and cook until softened, about 5 minutes.
3. Stir in the garlic-infused oil and dried thyme. Cook for another 1-2 minutes.
4. Add the sliced zucchini, diced potatoes, and chicken broth. Bring to a boil.
5. Reduce heat and simmer for 20-25 minutes until the vegetables are tender.
6. Puree the soup using an immersion blender or in batches using a regular blender until smooth.
7. Stir in the lactose-free milk and heat through.
8. Garnish with fresh chives before serving.

Nutrition Info per Serving

- Calories: 220
- Protein: 6g
- Carbohydrates: 30g
- Fat: 8g
- Fiber: 5g

Serves

- 4

Cooking Time

- 35 minutes

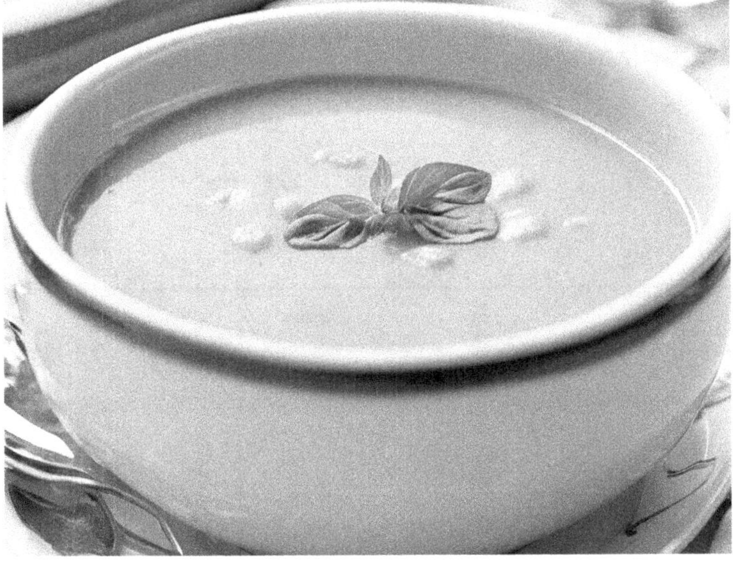

13. Clam Soup

Ingredients

- 2 cups clams, chopped (fresh or canned)
- 4 cups low-sodium chicken broth
- 1 cup lactose-free milk
- 2 potatoes, diced
- 1 onion, diced
- 2 celery stalks, sliced
- 2 tablespoons olive oil
- 1 tablespoon garlic-infused oil
- 1 teaspoon dried thyme
- 1 bay leaf
- 1/4 cup fresh parsley, chopped (for garnish)

Instructions

1. In a large pot, heat olive oil over medium heat.
2. Add the diced onion and celery. Cook until softened, about 5 minutes.
3. Stir in the garlic-infused oil, dried thyme, and bay leaf. Cook for another 1-2 minutes.
4. Add the diced potatoes and chicken broth. Bring to a boil.
5. Reduce heat and simmer for 15-20 minutes until the potatoes are tender.
6. Add the clams and lactose-free milk, and cook for another 5 minutes until heated through.
7. Remove the bay leaf before serving.
8. Garnish with fresh parsley before serving.

Nutrition Info per Serving

- Calories: 250
- Protein: 18g
- Carbohydrates: 28g
- Fat: 10g
- Fiber: 4g

Serves

- 4

Cooking Time

- 30 minutes

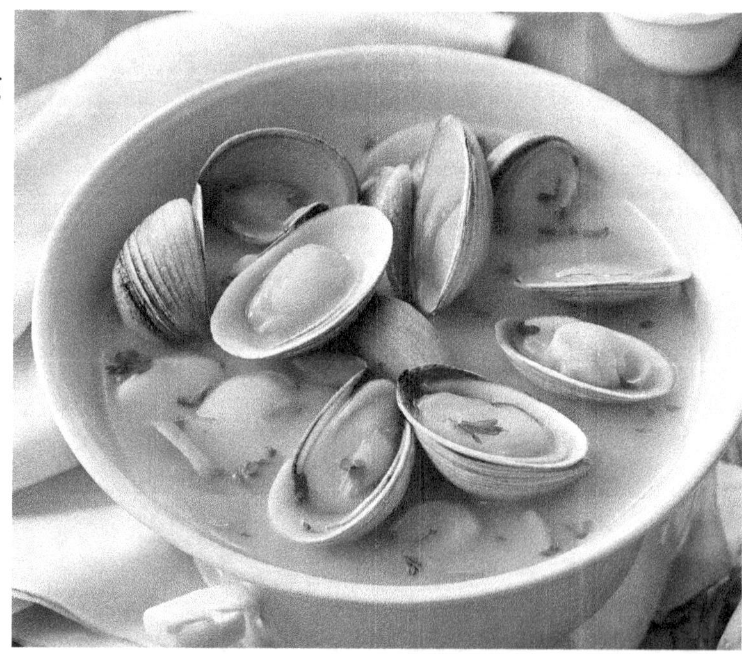

14. Thai Green Curry with Chicken

Ingredients

- 1 pound boneless, skinless chicken breast, cut into bite-sized pieces
- 1 onion, diced
- 1 red bell pepper, sliced
- 1 zucchini, sliced
- 1 cup green beans, trimmed
- 4 cups low-sodium chicken broth
- 1 can coconut milk
- 2 tablespoons green curry paste (ensure it's low FODMAP)
- 1 tablespoon garlic-infused oil
- 2 tablespoons olive oil
- 1 tablespoon fish sauce (ensure it's low FODMAP)
- 1 tablespoon lime juice
- 1/4 cup fresh basil, chopped (for garnish)

Instructions

1. In a large pot, heat olive oil over medium heat.
2. Add the chicken pieces and cook until browned, about 5-7 minutes. Remove and set aside.
3. In the same pot, add the diced onion and garlic-infused oil. Cook until softened, about 5 minutes.
4. Stir in the green curry paste and cook for another 1-2 minutes.
5. Add the red bell pepper, zucchini, and green beans. Cook for 3-4 minutes.
6. Return the chicken to the pot and add the chicken broth and coconut milk. Bring to a boil.
7. Reduce heat and simmer for 15-20 minutes until the chicken is cooked through and the vegetables are tender.
8. Stir in the fish sauce and lime juice.
9. Garnish with fresh basil before serving.

Nutrition Info per Serving

- Calories: 350
- Protein: 28g
- Carbohydrates: 18g
- Fat: 20g
- Fiber: 4g

Serves

- 4

Cooking Time

- 40 minutes

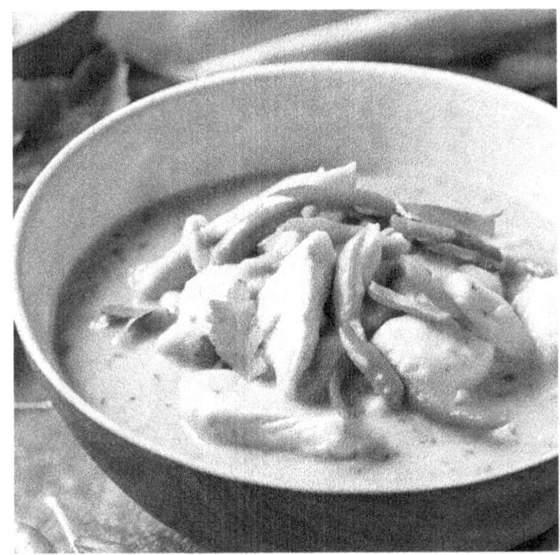

15. Squash and Carrot Stew

Ingredients

- 2 cups butternut squash, peeled and cubed
- 2 cups carrots, sliced
- 1 onion, diced
- 4 cups vegetable broth (low sodium)
- 1 cup coconut milk (canned)
- 2 tablespoons olive oil
- 1 tablespoon garlic-infused oil
- 1 teaspoon ground cumin
- 1/2 teaspoon ground coriander
- 1/4 cup fresh cilantro, chopped (for garnish)

Instructions

1. In a large pot, heat olive oil over medium heat.
2. Add the diced onion and cook until softened, about 5 minutes.
3. Stir in the garlic-infused oil, ground cumin, and ground coriander. Cook for another 1-2 minutes.
4. Add the cubed butternut squash, sliced carrots, and vegetable broth. Bring to a boil.
5. Reduce heat and simmer for 25-30 minutes until the vegetables are tender.
6. Puree half of the stew using an immersion blender or in batches using a regular blender until smooth, then return to the pot.
7. Stir in the coconut milk and heat through.
8. Garnish with fresh cilantro before serving.

Nutrition Info per Serving

- Calories: 280
- Protein: 4g
- Carbohydrates: 38g
- Fat: 14g
- Fiber: 8g

Serves

- 4

Cooking Time

- 40 minutes

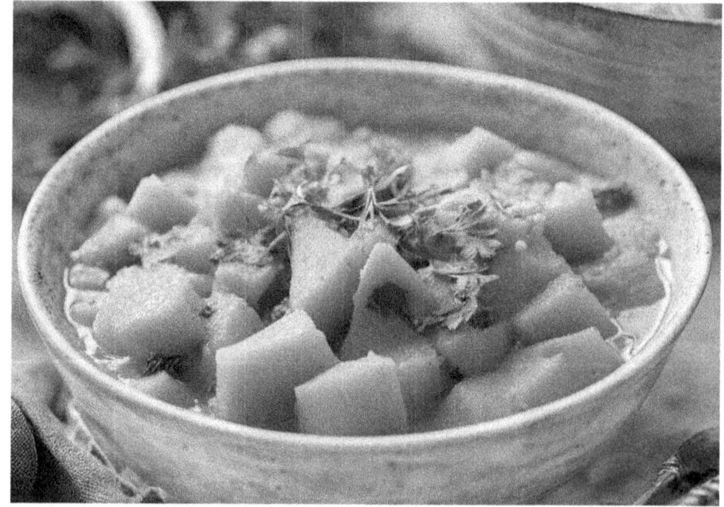

8-WEEK MEAL PLAN

Week 1
Monday:
- Breakfast: Sweet Potato Toast
- Lunch: Chicken and Broccoli Stir-Fry
- Dinner: Beef Shepherd's Pie

Tuesday:
- Breakfast: Buckwheat Pancakes
- Lunch: Tuna Nicoise Salad
- Dinner: Spicy Chicken Stew

Wednesday:
- Breakfast: Egg Muffins
- Lunch: Pork and Chive Dumplings
- Dinner: Baked Trout

Thursday:
- Breakfast: Lemon Garlic Turkey Cutlets
- Lunch: Chicken Tortilla Soup
- Dinner: Pork Schnitzel

Friday:
- Breakfast: Smoked Salmon Breakfast Plate
- Lunch: Turkey Stuffed Bell Peppers
- Dinner: Grilled Swordfish

Saturday:
- Breakfast: Raspberry Smoothie Bowl
- Lunch: Quinoa Vegetable Stew
- Dinner: Beef Carpaccio

Sunday:
- Breakfast: Almond Flour Muffins
- Lunch: Vegetable and Lentil Stew
- Dinner: Chicken Cacciatore

Week 2
Monday:
- Breakfast: Rice-Based Cereal
- Lunch: Shrimp and Grits
- Dinner: Pork Stew

Tuesday:
- Breakfast: Almond Porridge
- Lunch: Salmon and Spinach Quiche
- Dinner: White Fish Stew

Wednesday:
- Breakfast: Grilled Plantains
- Lunch: Broccoli Soup
- Dinner: Beef Ragout

Thursday:
- Breakfast: Strawberry Oat Bars
- Lunch: Leek and Potato Soup
- Dinner: Pork Pad Thai

Friday:
- Breakfast: Pineapple and Cucumber Salad
- Lunch: Clam Chowder
- Dinner: Seared Scallops

Saturday:
- Breakfast: Protein Shake
- Lunch: Zucchini Soup
- Dinner: Roast Turkey

Sunday:
- Breakfast: Stir-Fried Tempeh
- Lunch: Sauerkraut Soup
- Dinner: Chicken Paella

Week 3

Monday:
- Breakfast: Potato and Carrot Rosti
- Lunch: Thai Green Curry with Chicken
- Dinner: Baked Haddock

Tuesday:
- Breakfast: Savory Porridge
- Lunch: Spicy Chicken Stew
- Dinner: Grilled Mackerel

Wednesday:
- Breakfast: Homemade Hash Browns
- Lunch: Clam Soup
- Dinner: Pork Schnitzel

Thursday:
- Breakfast: Pumpkin Pancakes
- Lunch: Quinoa Vegetable Stew
- Dinner: Chicken Shawarma

Friday:
- Breakfast: Buckwheat Crepes
- Lunch: Sweet Potato and Ginger Soup
- Dinner: Halibut Steaks

Saturday:
- Breakfast: Smoked Herring
- Lunch: Chicken Tortilla Soup
- Dinner: Pork Piccata

Sunday:
- Breakfast: Savory Porridge
- Lunch: Broccoli Soup
- Dinner: Beef Bourguignon

Week 4

Monday:
- Breakfast: Turkey and Spinach Meatloaf
- Lunch: Squash and Carrot Stew
- Dinner: Grilled Chicken Skewers

Tuesday:
- Breakfast: Seared Scallops
- Lunch: Lemon Baked Sole
- Dinner: Irish Stew

Wednesday:
- Breakfast: Cauliflower and Turmeric Soup
- Lunch: Chicken Cacciatore
- Dinner: Pork Fajitas

Thursday:
- Breakfast: Pesto Shrimp Pasta
- Lunch: Chicken and Vegetable Kebabs
- Dinner: Pork Paillard

Friday:
- Breakfast: Raspberry Smoothie Bowl
- Lunch: Tuna Nicoise Salad
- Dinner: Pork Stew

Saturday:
- Breakfast: Protein Shake
- Lunch: Chicken Tortilla Soup
- Dinner: Sea Bass en Papillote

Sunday:
- Breakfast: Quinoa Porridge
- Lunch: Clam Soup
- Dinner: Beef Yakitori

Week 5

Monday:
- Breakfast: Sweet Potato Toast
- Lunch: Chicken and Broccoli Stir-Fry
- Dinner: Beef Shepherd's Pie

Tuesday:
- Breakfast: Egg Muffins
- Lunch: Tuna Nicoise Salad
- Dinner: Spicy Chicken Stew

Wednesday:
- Breakfast: Lemon Garlic Turkey Cutlets
- Lunch: Pork and Chive Dumplings
- Dinner: Baked Trout

Thursday:
- Breakfast: Smoked Salmon Breakfast Plate
- Lunch: Chicken Tortilla Soup
- Dinner: Pork Schnitzel

Friday:
- Breakfast: Raspberry Smoothie Bowl
- Lunch: Turkey Stuffed Bell Peppers
- Dinner: Grilled Swordfish

Saturday:
- Breakfast: Almond Flour Muffins
- Lunch: Quinoa Vegetable Stew
- Dinner: Beef Carpaccio

Sunday:
- Breakfast: Rice-Based Cereal
- Lunch: Vegetable and Lentil Stew
- Dinner: Chicken Cacciatore

Week 6

Monday:
- Breakfast: Almond Porridge
- Lunch: Shrimp and Grits
- Dinner: Pork Stew

Tuesday:
- Breakfast: Pineapple and Cucumber Salad
- Lunch: Salmon and Spinach Quiche
- Dinner: White Fish Stew

Wednesday:
- Breakfast: Grilled Plantains
- Lunch: Broccoli Soup
- Dinner: Beef Ragout

Thursday:
- Breakfast: Strawberry Oat Bars
- Lunch: Leek and Potato Soup
- Dinner: Pork Pad Thai

Friday:
- Breakfast: Protein Shake
- Lunch: Clam Chowder
- Dinner: Seared Scallops

Saturday:
- Breakfast: Stir-Fried Tempeh
- Lunch: Zucchini Soup
- Dinner: Roast Turkey

Sunday:
- Breakfast: Potato and Carrot Rosti
- Lunch: Sauerkraut Soup
- Dinner: Chicken Paella

Week 7

Monday:
- Breakfast: Homemade Hash Browns
- Lunch: Thai Green Curry with Chicken
- Dinner: Baked Haddock

Tuesday:
- Breakfast: Pumpkin Pancakes
- Lunch: Spicy Chicken Stew
- Dinner: Grilled Mackerel

Wednesday:
- Breakfast: Smoked Herring
- Lunch: Clam Soup
- Dinner: Pork Schnitzel

Thursday:
- Breakfast: Cauliflower and Turmeric Soup
- Lunch: Quinoa Vegetable Stew
- Dinner: Chicken Shawarma

Friday:

- Breakfast: Savory Porridge
- Lunch: Sweet Potato and Ginger Soup
- Dinner: Halibut Steaks

Saturday:

- Breakfast: Buckwheat Crepes
- Lunch: Chicken Tortilla Soup
- Dinner: Pork Piccata

Sunday:

- Breakfast: Savory Porridge
- Lunch: Broccoli Soup
- Dinner: Beef Bourguignon

Week 8

Monday:

- Breakfast: Turkey and Spinach Meatloaf
- Lunch: Squash and Carrot Stew
- Dinner: Grilled Chicken Skewers

Tuesday:

- Breakfast: Seared Scallops
- Lunch: Lemon Baked Sole
- Dinner: Irish Stew

Wednesday:

- Breakfast: Cauliflower and Turmeric Soup
- Lunch: Chicken Cacciatore
- Dinner: Pork Fajitas

Thursday:

- Breakfast: Pesto Shrimp Pasta
- Lunch: Chicken and Vegetable Kebabs
- Dinner: Pork Paillard

Friday:

- Breakfast: Raspberry Smoothie Bowl
- Lunch: Tuna Nicoise Salad
- Dinner: Pork Stew

Saturday:

- Breakfast: Protein Shake
- Lunch: Chicken Tortilla Soup
- Dinner: Sea Bass en Papillote

Sunday:

- Breakfast: Quinoa Porridge
- Lunch: Clam Soup
- Dinner: Beef Yakitori

WEEKLY MEAL PLANNER + WORKBOOK

	BREAKFAST	LUNCH	DINNER	SNACKS
MONDAY				
TUESDAY				
WEDNESDAY				
THURSDAY				
FRIDAY				
SATURDAY				
SUNDAY				

HOW WOULD YOU DESCRIBE YOUR CURRENT SYMPTOMS RELATED TO ENDOMETRIOSIS? LIST ANY PAIN, DISCOMFORT, OR DIGESTIVE ISSUES YOU EXPERIENCE REGULARLY.

WEEKLY MEAL PLANNER + WORKBOOK

	BREAKFAST	LUNCH	DINNER	SNACKS
MONDAY				
TUESDAY				
WEDNESDAY				
THURSDAY				
FRIDAY				
SATURDAY				
SUNDAY				

WHAT DOES YOUR TYPICAL DAILY DIET LOOK LIKE? INCLUDE MEALS, SNACKS, AND BEVERAGES.

WEEKLY MEAL PLANNER + WORKBOOK

	BREAKFAST	LUNCH	DINNER	SNACKS
MONDAY				
TUESDAY				
WEDNESDAY				
THURSDAY				
FRIDAY				
SATURDAY				
SUNDAY				

CAN YOU IDENTIFY ANY SPECIFIC FOODS OR MEALS THAT SEEM TO WORSEN YOUR ENDOMETRIOSIS SYMPTOMS? DESCRIBE THESE INSTANCES.

WEEKLY MEAL PLANNER + WORKBOOK

	BREAKFAST	LUNCH	DINNER	SNACKS
MONDAY				
TUESDAY				
WEDNESDAY				
THURSDAY				
FRIDAY				
SATURDAY				
SUNDAY				

KEEP A FOOD DIARY FOR ONE WEEK, NOTING EVERYTHING YOU EAT AND DRINK, ALONG WITH ANY SYMPTOMS YOU EXPERIENCE. HOW DO YOUR SYMPTOMS CORRELATE WITH YOUR DIET?

WEEKLY MEAL PLANNER + WORKBOOK

	BREAKFAST	LUNCH	DINNER	SNACKS
MONDAY				
TUESDAY				
WEDNESDAY				
THURSDAY				
FRIDAY				
SATURDAY				
SUNDAY				

WHY DO YOU WANT TO TRY THE LOW FODMAP DIET? WHAT ARE YOUR MAIN GOALS IN FOLLOWING THIS DIET PLAN?

WEEKLY MEAL PLANNER + WORKBOOK

	BREAKFAST	LUNCH	DINNER	SNACKS
MONDAY				
TUESDAY				
WEDNESDAY				
THURSDAY				
FRIDAY				
SATURDAY				
SUNDAY				

WHAT DO YOU KNOW ABOUT THE LOW FODMAP DIET? LIST ANY FOODS YOU KNOW ARE ALLOWED AND THOSE THAT ARE RESTRICTED.

WEEKLY MEAL PLANNER + WORKBOOK

	BREAKFAST	LUNCH	DINNER	SNACKS
MONDAY				
TUESDAY				
WEDNESDAY				
THURSDAY				
FRIDAY				
SATURDAY				
SUNDAY				

WHAT CHALLENGES DO YOU FORESEE WHEN GROCERY SHOPPING FOR LOW FODMAP FOODS? HOW CAN YOU OVERCOME THESE CHALLENGES?

....

....

....

....

....

....

WEEKLY MEAL PLANNER + WORKBOOK

	BREAKFAST	LUNCH	DINNER	SNACKS
MONDAY				
TUESDAY				
WEDNESDAY				
THURSDAY				
FRIDAY				
SATURDAY				
SUNDAY				

WHAT ARE SOME WAYS YOU CAN PREPARE AND COOK LOW FODMAP MEALS TO ENSURE THEY ARE BOTH TASTY AND NUTRITIOUS?

WEEKLY MEAL PLANNER + WORKBOOK

	BREAKFAST	LUNCH	DINNER	SNACKS
MONDAY				
TUESDAY				
WEDNESDAY				
THURSDAY				
FRIDAY				
SATURDAY				
SUNDAY				

HOW CAN YOU MANAGE YOUR DIET WHEN EATING OUT AT RESTAURANTS OR SOCIAL EVENTS? LIST STRATEGIES YOU CAN USE.

WEEKLY MEAL PLANNER + WORKBOOK

	BREAKFAST	LUNCH	DINNER	SNACKS
MONDAY				
TUESDAY				
WEDNESDAY				
THURSDAY				
FRIDAY				
SATURDAY				
SUNDAY				

HOW MUCH WATER DO YOU DRINK DAILY? DO YOU THINK YOUR HYDRATION HABITS AFFECT YOUR SYMPTOMS?

....

....

....

....

....

....

WEEKLY MEAL PLANNER + WORKBOOK

	BREAKFAST	LUNCH	DINNER	SNACKS
MONDAY				
TUESDAY				
WEDNESDAY				
THURSDAY				
FRIDAY				
SATURDAY				
SUNDAY				

REFLECT ON A TIME WHEN YOU SUCCESSFULLY MADE A SIGNIFICANT LIFESTYLE CHANGE. HOW CAN YOU APPLY THE LESSONS LEARNED FROM THAT EXPERIENCE TO STARTING THE LOW FODMAP DIET?

Scan the QR code below to get a surprise bonus!